The Woman
Who Revolutionised
Nurses' Training

The Woman
Who Revolutionised
Nurses' Training

The Life and Career of Rebecca Strong

Judith Vallely

PEN & SWORD
HISTORY

AN IMPRINT OF PEN & SWORD BOOKS LTD.
YORKSHIRE - PHILADELPHIA

First published in Great Britain in 2024 by
Pen & Sword History
An imprint of
Pen & Sword Books Ltd
Yorkshire - Philadelphia

ISBN 978 1 39906 165 0

A CIP catalogue record for this book is available from the British Library.

Typeset in INDIA by IMPEC eSolutions
Printed and bound in England by CPI (UK) Ltd.

Pen & Sword Books Limited incorporates the imprints of Archaeology, Atlas,
Aviation, Battleground, Digital, Discovery, Family History, Fiction, History,
Local, Local History, Maritime, Military, Military Classics, Politics, Select,
Transport, True Crime, After the Battle, Air World, Claymore Press, Frontline
Publishing, Leo Cooper, Remember When, Seaforth Publishing, The Praetorian
Press, Wharncliffe Books, Wharncliffe Local History, Wharncliffe Transport,
Wharncliffe True Crime and White Owl.

For a complete list of Pen & Sword titles please contact

PEN & SWORD BOOKS LIMITED
47 Church Street, Barnsley, South Yorkshire, S70 2AS, England
E-mail: enquiries@pen-and-sword.co.uk
Website: www.pen-and-sword.co.uk

or

PEN AND SWORD BOOKS
1950 Lawrence Rd, Havertown, PA 19083, USA
E-mail: uspen-and-sword@casematepublishers.com
Website: www.penandswordbooks.com

MIX
Paper | Supporting
responsible forestry
FSC
www.fsc.org   FSC® C013604

Contents

Introduction: 'A Very Troublesome Woman'

When it comes to the career and life of Rebecca Strong, there are many fascinating details. She was the first ever nurse to take a patient's temperature – using a thermometer – which in those days was an awkward instrument, shaped like a shepherd's crook around 2ft long. For this she was scolded, as at that time it was seen as a right which could only be performed by doctors.

Strong controversially introduced a 'no drinking' rule at a time when nurses would have beer on duty. She resigned from a key post after hospital management failed to meet her requests for a proper nurses' home. She met Italian dictator Mussolini and had a white feather given to her by a Native American chief at a jamboree held in her honour.

I first came across Strong when I was researching my book *Struggle and Suffrage in Glasgow: Women's Lives and the Fight for Equality*, looking at the inspirational women of my home city and their quest for equal rights and improvements in all areas of society. A brief delve into snippets of her life intrigued me: being widowed at an early age; training with Florence Nightingale; introducing revolutionary new methods during her time as matron at Glasgow Royal Infirmary; working with some of the most eminent doctors of the age; and continuing to travel all over the world during retirement until her death at 100.

The biggest surprise was that her name is largely unknown. Despite her amazing life, like so many women of her time, it has long been overlooked. The names of eminent doctors of the Victorian era – Joseph Lister, William Macewen, Alexander Fleming – have rightly lived on in the history books as the pioneers of a time when crucial advances in medicine were being made, including the founding of antiseptic surgery and breakthroughs in surgical techniques.

What is less widely known is a revolution was also underway in the field of nursing, which transformed caring for the sick from a job seen as being carried out by untrained, incompetent drunk women, into a role which relied on an educated and trained workforce. Florence Nightingale, of course, is a name which has been recognised for generations as the founder of modern nursing. However, the achievements of Strong in developing this work equally deserve to be celebrated and brought to a wider audience.

Her contributions have not gone entirely unnoticed, thanks to the dedication of the Friends of Glasgow Royal Infirmary, a charity which aims to celebrate the hospital's heritage and long history and has set up a dedicated museum. Despite undergoing many changes since it was founded in 1794 – including being rebuilt in the early twentieth century – the hospital still stands in a prominent position in the city near the cathedral and treats thousands of patients every year. This was the main place where Strong was to develop and implement her ideas for a programme of education for nursing. There is a display dedicated to her in the Friends of Glasgow Royal Infirmary Museum, and at the opening event in May 2022, her great great-grandson David Geyer gave a speech as he formally opened it:

> I'm sure if I said to any one of you, oh I knew a lady quite well, she was born in 1843, I think your initial reaction would be 'don't be ridiculous'. But not only did I know Rebecca Strong, or in fact what we have always known as Granny Strong, because she was my father's granny ... you're actually looking at somebody who did know Rebecca Strong really quite well, and not only just. I was 15 years old when she died and we didn't see much of her in the latter years because the war was on and I couldn't travel. But I met her on a number of occasions and she was a very formidable woman.[1]

He also recounted his memories of meeting Strong when she was in her nineties, in an interview given at the time of the opening of the museum:

> I remember her coming to see us in Wakefield, where we lived, in the summer of 1939, not long before the war broke out. I was 10. We went to the railway station to meet her and you can imagine this station, mid-morning, not much colour – and then out steps Rebecca

Strong from the carriage, dressed up to the nines in the most beautiful clothing. She strode towards us, fit as a fiddle aged 95. She was quite amazing.[2]

However, he also said the family did not really talk about her career and status as a 'famous nurse':

It wasn't a subject brought up in conversation. We're all very pleased she's being remembered. It would be a pity if she disappeared without someone singing her praises.

Strong's formidable character was clearly key in forging the way ahead when it came to improving the standards of care and training of nurses, often resulting in clashes with hospital authorities. Speaking about her efforts to have a proper nurses' home built, she summed it up in what has become one of the most famous quotes associated with her: 'I am afraid I was a very troublesome woman. As soon as one step was taken I proposed another.'[3]

However, as this book will explore, it was precisely this determined spirit which means she is now widely regarded as the founder of modern nursing in Scotland:

Her unique contribution to nurse education was to initiate the block apprenticeship training program which would soon become commonplace throughout schools of nursing everywhere, i.e. short bursts of periodic theoretical input within the school of nursing followed by periods of nursing practice. She was also credited with introducing the concept of the preliminary training school (PTS) which persists around the world in one form or another in schools of nursing to this day.[4]

As far as I have been able to establish, until now there has been no biography of Strong – although there are several articles and chapters within books examining her work and life. Modest about her achievements, she only wrote a short memoir of her own life when she was in her eighties, leaving many gaps to be filled in.

The eightieth anniversary of Strong's death will take place in 2024, as well as the hundredth anniversary of the death of Sir William Macewen, the famous Scottish surgeon who, as we shall see, both encouraged her work and also acknowledged the role it had supporting his own pioneering breakthroughs in surgery.

It is only right that the life and lasting legacy of both these remarkable pioneers should be celebrated.

Chapter One

Old, Weak, Drunken, Stupid: The Stereotype of Early Nurses

She was a fat old woman, this Mrs Gamp, with a husky voice and a moist eye, which she had a remarkable power of turning up, and only showing the white of it. Having very little neck, it cost her some trouble to look over herself, if one may say so, at those to whom she talked. She wore a very rusty black gown, rather the worse for snuff, and a shawl and bonnet to correspond. In these dilapidated articles of dress she had, on principle, arrayed herself, time out of mind, on such occasions as the present; for this at once expressed a decent amount of veneration for the deceased, and invited the next of kin to present her with a fresher suit of weeds; an appeal so frequently successful, that the very fetch and ghost of Mrs Gamp, bonnet and all, might be seen hanging up, any hour in the day, in at least a dozen of the second-hand clothes shops about Holborn. The face of Mrs Gamp – the nose in particular – was somewhat red and swollen, and it was difficult to enjoy her society without becoming conscious of a smell of spirits. Like most persons who have attained to great eminence in their profession, she took to hers very kindly; insomuch that, setting aside her natural predilections as a woman, she went to a lying-in or a laying-out with equal zest and relish.[1]

This description of Sarah Gamp, the nurse depicted by Charles Dickens in the novel *Martin Chuzzlewit*, published in 1844, is a far cry from the professional staff we know of today, who undertake years of training and qualifications to enable them to work on the wards. Yet the author is said to have based her on a real nurse. The image of an untrained, incompetent drunk was the stereotype of nurses during the eighteenth and first half of the nineteenth century. There is debate over to what extent this was true – some critics have pointed out that Dickens supported the medical fraternity, who wanted complete control over health and caring, while others note the suggestion that the characterisation of Mrs Gamp could have been reflective of attempts to undermine a female-led working-class nursing movement in favour of a nursing workforce dominated by the male medical world.

This was a discussion raised in the pages of *The Nursing Record* journal, around half a century after Dickens published his work, in an article considering how the profession had changed in that time. The nurse of 1896, it noted, is 'absolutely a different creature from her immediate predecessor – different in manner, in intellect, in appearance, and, above all, in her training – that it is difficult for the younger generation to realise what even their immediate predecessors were like'.[2] The article said a look back at some of the 'old-world nurses' finds that they certainly 'did not rank very high in public esteem':

Imagine anyone now a days writing as 'Marian' does in the *The Woman in White*: 'Professional Nurses, proverbially as cruel a set of women as any to be found in England'. If that statement were published in a novel now what a hubbub would ensue! ... And yet as far as I know, this remark has never been criticised before, in a public at least, which in itself throws a curious sidelight on the differences which have come about in the position of Nurses since Wilkie Collins published his great masterpiece.[3]

Some more portrayals of nurses in literature are examined – including Mrs Gamp who is described as 'so repulsive, with her drink and her vulgarity, her ignorance and toadyism'. Charlotte Brontë's depiction of Mrs Horsfall in her novel *Shirley*, published in 1849 after Jane Eyre, is also noted:

> Mrs Horsfall is really an appalling female, described in one place as 'a sort of giantess'; in another as 'no woman, but a dragon', and again as 'that ogress'; yet, we are told, she was the best Nurse on the staff of an apparently flourishing country surgeon. We do not wonder to read that her patient 'hated the site of her rough bulk, and dreaded the touch of her hard hands'; but we do wonder a good deal at his recovery, when we are told that when he was bad 'she shook him'.

However, it does go on to say these portrayals in fictions are 'sweeping assertions', noting that 'there can be no large body of women (and Nurses must always have been fairly numerous) without there being some true and gentle ones amongst them.'[4]

Yet, what is true is that no formal educational training for nurses existed in the nineteenth century, although some hospital doctors offered tuition on the 'basic elements of care' to their nursing staff.[5] And while a stereotype may have existed, records suggest there was indeed often some truth in the portrayal of nurses at this time.

Lothian Health Services Archive holds the diary of Angélique Lucille Pringle, who trained with Nightingale. It covers a visit to the Royal Infirmary of Edinburgh (RIE) in November 1872, which contains her observations on these 'old school' nurses:

> Pringle makes mention of nurses being intoxicated. In one instance, a night nurse called Annie Fisher is caught asleep on the job. After many attempts to wake the nurse up, Mrs Barclay asks Fisher 'what about your patients, nurse?' Laughing, Fisher replies, 'Oh, I had nae mind o' them', which Pringle writes is a 'skillful epitome of the state of nursing'. After Pringle and Barclay wake up a day nurse to take charge of the ward, Annie Fisher follows the two women, enraged and screaming that she 'had seen a good many out and she would see us out too!'[6]

However, perhaps there is little surprise that nurses did not have the best reputation, given that at the time they had to endure such poor working conditions:

The nurses at the RIE pre-1870s 'were poorly housed, ill-fed, underpaid and over-worked, and many of them were regarded as attendants and servants rather than nurses'. Shockingly, the night nurses' shifts were extraordinarily long – they would come on duty at 11 o'clock at night and their shift would not end until 5 p.m. the next day! Their shifts were so long because, after completing their nightly nursing duties, they would still have to make breakfast and clean the dishes and wards and give patients their food.[7]

Researchers have noted that by no means were all nurses of this time drunk and poorly educated, and many showed incredible devotion to their job. For example, during the cholera epidemic of 1854, the norm was to work without respite:

Sisters showed no concern for themselves, one nurse died after having refused to report her diarrhoea and go off duty, another developed cholera but eventually recovered.[8]

The records also show the sacrifice many others made for their job, with a high sickness and death rate among nurses:

During the first 50 years at the Middlesex Hospital, no less than 12 nurses died out of an average complement of eight while at St Bartholomew's in the 1850s–1860s,

27 nurses died of 'fever'. The cause of death is seldom recorded, but as Florence Nightingale was later to point out, hospitals themselves were a source of infection and did the patient more harm than good.[9]

The idea of drinking on duty would be seen as outrageous today, but it must be remembered this was also an era in which water was contaminated and tea was taxed at 100 per cent – with 'beer and porter the main drinks available to the poor':

> Furthermore, in the absence of analgesics – aspirin was not available until 1899 – alcohol and laudanum were the only means of assuaging physical pain or mental distress.[10]

The perception of nursing was to change thanks to one of the most acclaimed women in history – Florence Nightingale. Famously known as the 'Lady with the Lamp', her efforts in looking after of sick and wounded soldiers during the Crimean War has become the epitome of a caring nurse. But her achievements went far beyond this, helping to transform the haphazard occupation associated with the like of Mrs Gamp into a respectable career.

Nightingale described the state of nursing before reform as for 'those who were too old, too weak, too drunken, too dirty, too stupid or too bad to do anything else'. Indeed, her decision to become a nurse provoked consternation among her family, who had a background as wealthy landowners. At the time, it was not seen as a suitable job for a young lady.

She became known as an authority of nursing after being appointed the superintendent for the Institute for the Care of Sick Gentlewomen in Harley Street, London in early 1853. The following year, when Britain became involved in the Crimean War, the reports from war correspondents – who had been allowed to be present on the battlefield for the first time – highlighted the inadequate provision of care for injured and sick soldiers. In response to an outpouring of anger, Nightingale was asked to help and within days enlisted a group of volunteer nurses to go to the war zone, where her reputation was made as she worked tirelessly to tend to her patients.

Her reputation as the Lady with the Lamp was born as she conducted her night-time rounds of the hospital carrying a simple Turkish paper concertina lantern. The wounded men began to call her the 'Angel of the Crimea' and would kiss her shadow as she walked by the beds. This adoration soon spread to the British public at home, following the publication of a pen and ink drawing of her carrying a lamp on her ward round in *The Illustrated London News* in 1855.[11]

However, she became gravely ill after contracting Crimean fever – a bacterial infection now known as brucellosis, which causes symptoms including fever, nausea, loss of appetite, sweating, headaches, extreme tiredness and joint pain. Antibiotic treatments were not available at this time and, while she recovered, the toll on her health continued for the rest of her life.

When she returned home after the war in 1856 she inevitably sailed out of the pages of history and into legend.[12]

Yet Nightingale's achievements as a nurse were not just about her caring nature, as is sometimes popularly portrayed. She had the advantage of an education, including in mathematics, and after returning home from Crimea, analysed data collected on the patients along with William Farr, one of the leading statisticians of the time:

> While she was aware of the high death rate at the hospital in Scutari, she had attributed it to poor nutrition, suboptimal treatment and delayed transfer to hospital from the battlefront. It was only when Farr helped her to analyse the data that she realised that more lives could have been saved if she had had a greater focus on basic sanitation. One of Nightingale's first books, *Notes on Matters Affecting Health, Efficiency, and Hospital Administration of the British Army* (1858), used statistical methods to compare the deaths rates of the army in peacetime with the civilian rate. Together with Farr, she showed that mortality was due to hospital conditions and concluded that 'our soldiers are enlisted to die in barracks.'[13]

These ideas were expanded upon in Nightingale's *Notes on Nursing*, which was published the following year in 1859.

She wrote extensive descriptions of the ideal conditions for patients, such as the need for clean air, adequate ventilation and light, clean water and reducing unnecessary noise. She also noted that poor living conditions could result in increasing the risk of infections:

I have known cases of hospital pyaemia quite as severe in handsome private hospitals, and from the same cause, viz, foul air. Yet nobody learnt the lesson. Nobody learnt *anything* at all from it. They went on *thinking* – thinking that the sufferer had scratched his thumb, or that it was singular that 'all the servants' had 'whitlow' [infection of the finger] or that something was 'much about this year; there is always sickness in our house'. This is a favourite mode of thought – leading *not* to inquire what is the uniform cause of these general 'whitlow', but to stifle all inquiry. In what sense is 'sickness' being 'always there', a justification of its being 'there' at all?[14]

She went on to outline the cause of the hospital pyaemia (infection) being present in the house, giving an insight into poor standard of living conditions in even the more affluent households of the time:

It was that the sewer air from an ill-placed sink was carefully conducted into all the rooms by sedulously opening all the doors and closing all the passage windows. It was that the slops were emptied into the foot pans; – it was that the utensils were never properly rinsed; – it was the chamber crockery was rinsed with dirty water; – it was that the beds were never properly shaken, aired, picked to pieces or changed. It was that the carpets and curtains were always musty; – it was that the furniture was always dusty; it was that the papered walls were saturated with dirt – it was that the floors were never cleaned …

It was Nightingale's establishment of the first UK school of nursing which was to set the path and transform the way in which future generations who followed her career path would be trained. On the back of her heroic efforts in the war, a fund set up in Nightingale's name had collected the equivalent of nearly £6 million in today's money from members of the public and the armed forces by 1859. She decided to set up a dedicated school of nursing within St Thomas' Hospital in London as part of her campaign around the improvement nursing and healthcare. It was led by superintendent Sarah Wardroper, as she was too sick to run it herself, and was the first ever professional nursing school in the world:

The launch of the first nursing school in 1860 drew a line in the sand, finally overcoming nursing's former Sairy Gamp image and creating a new horizon where nursing would be respected as a professional career choice for women. However, formal nurse registration in Britain was still nearly 60 years away and Nightingale herself was not supportive of later campaigns to introduce statutory state registration for nurses. It should be stressed that during the early years of the Nightingale school the cohorts of probationers were not actually trained to nurse but rather they were trained to train others. These Nightingale disciples were poised to promote the Nightingale training methodology across the whole of the country and further afield into other countries such as America and Australia.[15]

A report in *The Nursing Record and Hospital World*, published three decades after the Nightingale School was set up, reflected on the positive changes it had brought:

It was the Crimean War, which, by its terrible exposure of Governmental incapacity and unreadiness, afforded the opportunity to Miss Florence Nightingale to initiate a national movement by the attention drawn to the value of nursing work in the care of our sick and wounded soldiers. Fortunately for this country, Miss Nightingale not only possessed the pecuniary means, but also the skilled knowledge which enabled her to devote the funds subscribed by a grateful nation in her honour and to initiate a definite system of nursing education. Indeed, the Nightingale School must always be regarded as the first serious and properly organized attempt to place the training of nurses upon a sound and scientific basis.[16]

Nightingale's remarkable contribution has ensured her name remains a famous one today. To mark the centenary year of her birth, the World Health Organization designated 2020 as the International Year of the Nurse and the Midwife. During the Covid pandemic of the same year, a network of treatment centres built to help the NHS in England cope with the anticipated pressures of the virus were known as Nightingale hospitals.

In Scotland, a similar facility set up in Glasgow brought the name of a less well-known nurse to the attention of the public – Louisa Jordan. Born in Maryhill, Glasgow, she was a First World War nurse who signed up to the war effort in December 1914 while working as a Queen's nurse in Fife. She died on active service in Serbia just a year later while with the Scottish Women's Hospitals for Foreign Services and is still commemorated each year in Serbia along with her colleagues.

Back in the nineteenth century, the ethos of the school of nursing that was set up at the St Thomas' Hospital by Nightingale started being spread by its first disciples. They may not have become as well known as Nightingale but they all made vital contributions to the foundations of modern nursing.

They included Linda Richards, who pioneered the establishment of nurse training schools across the USA; Lucy Osburn, who went to Sydney after enrolling at the Nightingale School and is now regarded as the founder of modern nursing in Australia; and Alice Fisher, who established a nurse training school at Philadelphia General Hospital.[17]

That list, of course, also included Rebecca Strong – whose life, work and contribution to nursing will be explored in the coming pages.

Chapter Two

Learning from Florence Nightingale

While Strong was to spend much of her later life and career in Scotland, she was born on 23 August 1843 in London as Rebecca Thorogood. Most accounts of her life often state that 'practically nothing' is known about her early years, but there are some intriguing details which shed light on her family and the circumstances which may have helped formed her formidable and resilient character:

> She was born at the Blue Boar in Aldgate, London, an inn kept by her late father who was also a coach proprietor. It is possible that her husband was a mathematical instrument maker, and that their short married life was spent in Liverpool since her husband is buried there, but he presumably died too young to make provision for her and the baby Anne Ellen. Her parents, too, died soon after and the widowed young Rebecca had to look about for some way to keep herself and her child.[1]

Other accounts have similarly sparse details of her early life, but her motivation to get into nursing is largely attributed to being widowed at a young age and having to find a way to support her young daughter:

> She married young and had one daughter before she was 20. Little is known about her husband other than his name, Strong, that he died within a couple of years of their marriage, and was buried in Liverpool. Shortly after becoming a widow, Rebecca decided to do something with her life and, through the influence of a close friend who was a midwife, she chose to take up nursing.[2]

In a fascinating talk on the life of Strong,[3] Dr Kate Stevens, of the Friends of Glasgow Royal Infirmary, provides some more details, including that by 1851 the Thorogood family was living in Broxbourne, Hertfordshire. She speculates that Strong's father, John, may have taken on another coaching inn and notes that in 1854 her mother Mary died, leaving Rebecca to be brought up by her older sisters from the age of just 11.

Just one month short of her twentieth birthday, on 19 July 1863, Rebecca married Andrew Robert Strong, an instrument maker the same age. In 1864, they had a daughter, Anne Ellen Strong. This account by Stevens also confirms the marriage was extremely short lived – by 1865, Rebecca was said to be widowed. But she raises the intriguing possibility that the death of her husband may not have actually happened:

> Now whilst widowhood was effectively her situation, there is evidence that her husband was not in fact dead,

just missing and in 1866 the same Andrew Robert Strong instrument maker married again, presumably bigamously as there's no record of divorce from Rebecca in existence. Regardless, he exits the life of both Rebecca and Anne at this point.[4]

Whatever the circumstances of Rebecca being left on her own, there is general agreement that the unexpected situation she found herself provided impetus for her to embark on a career. As Stevens says:

It is worth reflecting upon that had Rebecca not found herself a single parent with a need to provide for herself and her daughter, she might not have embarked upon the fruitful, productive and successful work which has proven so important to the world of nursing.[5]

Indeed, this is confirmed in an article in *The British Journal of Nursing* published in 1924, in which Strong provided some details of the reasons that led her to adopt nursing as a career, in the hope of encouraging others who commence their professional careers under 'disadvantages'. It noted:

Being left a widow at a very early age, and anxious to make her life of some use, after consultation with an intimate friend – Mrs Firth, a prominent midwife – she concluded to try nursing. A sidelight on the status of nursing in the 'sixties of the last century, is that it was the usual thing for women who wished to become nurses to enter hospitals as scrubbers and work their way up. By this time, however, Miss Nightingale had established the Nightingale Training School at St Thomas' Hospital, where she had found Mrs Wardroper as Matron with advanced ideas and quietly working towards reformation, and, in certain wards, ladies, who had been given the title of 'Sister', were made directly responsible to the Physicians and Surgeons in charge of them.

From Mr Baggally, the then Governor, from Mrs Wardroper, and from one of the Sisters who had been amongst the first to take up the new work, Mrs Strong learnt something to its intention, and decided to enter the Nightingale Training School at St Thomas' Hospital.[6]

In June 1867, Strong was received as a probationer in the Nightingale School at the age of 24. In her short memoir, *Reminiscences*, published much later in her life in 1935, Strong recounted what she found on arrival at the hospital – including an emphasis on the 'good character' of the nurses being employed there. This was essential to ensure that the initiative being pioneered by Nightingale was not put at risk of criticism by members of the medical profession:

Women under the name of 'scrubber' were engaged to do the rougher work of the wards, and others of a better class were induced to act as nurses, under the superintendence of the sisters. A greater intelligence was then brought to bear upon the work, only women of good character being employed. This was a great advance which Miss Nightingale recognised, and made arrangements with the authorities for a certain number of pupils to be received, each to have a cubicle for sleeping and a common dining-room with a neat appointed table was also provided; at least that was what I found on entering the Nightingale School in 1867.[7]

At the time it was set up, the nurses' school was revolutionary – but looking back decades later Rebecca recounts that 'very little' was expected from the probationers because progress was 'slow' with regards to organised teaching. Perhaps this recollection serves to show just how far training had developed by the time she was writing her memoirs.

She also highlighted this in another interview, saying that by the end of the first year, it was assumed a nurse would have picked up enough knowledge to be able to pioneer work in any other hospitals to which they were sent:

Theoretical instruction was almost *nil*, which was a great disadvantage, the more enterprising had recourse to medical books.[8]

She notes in *Reminiscences*, however, that some principles were 'well ingrained' during her time at St Thomas' Hospital – including 'kindness, watchfulness, cleanliness and guarding against bedsores' and there were a few 'stray lectures':

One I remember especially, I think it was on the Chemistry of Life or some such title, it caused me to get a book on the subject, which I found most useful. There was a dummy on which to practise bandaging, and some lessons were given, also a skeleton, and some ancient medical books, one fortunately on Anatomy for those who attempted self-education. The more enterprising pupils provided themselves with something more modern, Hoblyn's dictionary [a nineteenth-century dictionary of medical and scientific terms] being a great favourite.[9]

Strong pointed out that while Nightingale herself had scrubbed floors and 'cleaned brasses' during her first experience of nursing – which took place during a three-month stint at The Deaconess Institute, Kaiserwerth, Germany[10] – she did not expect this of her own pupils; this made sure that the 'whole time on duty' was devoted to caring for patients. She described how some Latin abbreviations had to be learned so that directions on medicine bottles could be understood – adding that she did not find this difficult. But she noted that some aspects of care were initially strictly off limits for the probationers:

Temperature taking and chart keeping were medical students' work. I was once asked by a surgeon to take a temperature and, on being found by the sister in the act, was severely reprimanded for doing students' work, but from that time it gradually became the work of the nurse. The thermometer was in the form of a shepherd's crook, and had to be read in situ.

And there were also a few customs which would 'surprise the pupil of today', she noted:

On Saturday mornings two pupils were told … to make cakes for Sunday. Outdoor uniform was provided as well as in; the outdoor consisting of a shawl and bonnet worn over one's ordinary dress. A pupil was told … now and again to trim the bonnets: I had my turn, so you see we were supposed to be useful in various ways.

During Strong's time, a probationer entering the Nightingale School had to sign a contract for six years – but it was not the case that a nurse would have to remain at St Thomas' for the whole period. After one year of residence, it was expected that she would have gained sufficient knowledge to take her learning and knowledge about good nursing practices to other hospitals.

Strong described it as being a 'pioneer in other hospitals, at home and abroad' and noted that in her own year, Sydney Hospital in Australia was supplied with a matron and four nurses.[11] In 1868, she herself was sent to the new hospital at Winchester along with five other Nightingale nurses:

Miss Nightingale preferred to send several nurses together to a hospital, a group having a better chance of introducing reforms than one nurse on her own. At the Winchester Hospital, one nurse was assigned to each of the five wards and Rebecca Strong volunteered to do night duty, as she thought this work would be more interesting.[12]

Strong was said to have enjoyed the work and briefly described her time there in *Reminiscences*:

In the case of the new Winchester Hospital, the then Matron, Miss Freeman, was sent to the Nightingale School to see more modern methods of working a hospital, and on her return to Winchester six of us went with her as pioneers. There were five wards on three flats and six nurses, one day nurse to each ward, leaving one only for night; as I liked novelty, I volunteered for that duty. I had a central room from which sounds could be easily heard, and ward doors left open.

I am glad to say all went well. After a few weeks a woman without any knowledge of nursing was engaged to assist, which quickly proved unsatisfactory, and two additional nurses were appointed, which gave one nurse to each flat – a great relief.

However, after a year, Strong was recalled from Winchester to be sent to the new British army hospital at Netley, in Southampton. It no longer stands today, but was built in response to the Crimean

War, and on completion had the capacity to accommodate more than 1,000 patients in 138 wards.

Queen Victoria approved the plans to construct the hospital in 1856 and the Royal Victoria Hospital opened to patients in March 1863. Nightingale had been asked by the War Office to reorganise the nursing in the hospital and Strong noted that while an invalid at that time, she still gave each individual nurse an interview at her bedside 'exhorting us to take with us high ideals, and encouraging us to work on in hope – a privilege we all valued'.

In a letter of thanks to Nightingale, Strong expressed her gratitude for giving her two books – *The Heir of Radcliffe* and Scott's *Poetical Works*. She said she hoped she would have no cause for disappointment in giving her the appointment saying, 'I shall endeavour to throw all my energy into the work and to carry out your wishes in every way, hoping it will be successful.'[13]

An account in a newspaper around the time Strong was a nurse there gives an insight into life at Netley, describing how numerous men dressed in light-blue garments denoting that they were military invalids could be seen walking 'to and fro' on the esplanade or the pier, and that the building was the largest hospital in the world:

Netley Hospital is the headquarters of the invaliding of the Army, and although it is of so extensive a character, the building is at times comparatively full. Everything calculated to render the sick soldier comfortable, to restore him to health, or to benefit him if incurably diseased, has formed a matter for consideration, and many men have had good cause to remember their sojourn within its walls with gratitude. The climate, especially during the summer months, is delightful. Around stretches a magnificently wooded and picturesque country, while the constant refreshing sea breeze braces the enervated invalid, and the bustle of the river with the charming singing of the larks and nightingales (perhaps more plentiful and musical than in any part of England) arouses the dejected and hypochondriac. Reading-rooms, baths, recreation rooms, and out-door amusements are at the disposal of those who are capable of enjoying them, and during the winter months various entertainments have been produced within doors.[14]

Another report from 1871 gives information on the patients who were treated at the Royal Victoria Hospital during that year. It notes there were 2,747 admissions in total, with 1,826 arriving from India by the overland route and 161 by the Cape of Good Hope. The highest number in the hospital on any one day was 891 on 16 February and the lowest 37 on 18 December.[15]

Strong's own description of her time at the Netley in *Reminiscences* provides more insight into her work and those of her fellow nurses:

This was the beginning of Protestant 'Sisters' being employed in the British Army, and from this the present vast organisation has sprung. There was nominally an orderly attached to each ward, which contained about eight beds, to nurse the patients and clean the wards, but they were often taken away for relief work, such as coal carrying, etc. Each sister had from six to eight of these wards under her charge, and speedily found that the nursing must be done by herself: the distressing part was leaving anyone really ill at night to very scanty care. A special orderly could be had in emergencies, but the nursing was nil. When patients were received, it was from troopships of invalided men. It was not an easy matter for the medical officers to decide hastily who should go to the wards for treatment and who were ready for the convalescent side, the sea voyage having been beneficial to some. It was a few days before they were quite settled and, after the acute cases were finished with, the work became rather monotonous.

Her own words hardly give the impression that Strong enjoyed her time at Netley and this is backed by her decision in 1872 to leave and return to Winchester – which was technically a breach of her contract and almost led to her dismissal. Despite this, she did manage to go back to Winchester and finished her six years' service there.[16]

More than three decades after she became a probationer, Strong recounted her personal experience of learning to be a nurse, suggesting that it was not without challenges – and mistakes:

> Looking back upon my own early experience, and the work undertaken by me, without knowledge of the construction of the human frame, its functions, and the hygienic laws pertaining to the maintenance of health, and my ignorance of the leading features of disease, and inability to distinguish between healthy and unhealthy excretions, with the inevitable blunders arising therefrom (in fact learning through blubberers) which is not to be commended where risk to life is involved, I concluded that it was necessary to be acquainted with these matters before entering the Wards, to be instructed in the practical art of Nursing, as there is too much close study entailed in acquiring the elements of these things to admit of class being carried on simultaneously with ward work.[17]

These are ideas which she was to develop as her own career progressed and they formed the basis of her vision of the changes she wanted to see brought into nursing.

Chapter Three

Raising the Status of Nurses in Dundee

At the age of 31, Strong was appointed to her first senior position when she became matron of Dundee Royal Infirmary. She was hired to carry out a plan to establish a training school for nurses, instigated by Dr Robert Sinclair, who had been appointed medical superintendent of the hospital in 1873.

He was unhappy with the state of nursing at the infirmary, particularly among night staff, and after presenting a report on the unsatisfactory state of the nursing department he obtained the directors' approval to proceed with his plan to provide the first nursing training in Scotland, with special funds provided to set up the new venture.

This was an ideal opportunity for Strong to put some of the ideas that had been taking shape during her own years of training into practice – to improve the living conditions for nurses and also raise the status of the profession, with the work of caring for patients respected. This could be achieved, she believed, by providing a standard of education to the right candidates.

Meanwhile, Sinclair's ideas had already been partially carried out; accommodation had been built next to Dundee

Royal Infirmary to provide each nurse with a bedroom, improving the conditions in which they were working.

The hospital had been opened in 1798 and an account given in a lecture by a historian more than a century later[1] provides some interesting details on what life was like in those first years. A few pigs were kept by the apothecary – but the practice was stopped by the directors after the arrival of rats. The same directors were also surprised to find a colony of rabbits on one occasion, while the matron – who is not named – sometimes had to be told to keep her hens 'under better control'.

The first person to be admitted was William Dove, a joiner from Monikie, who was kept in for a fortnight and then sent home with 'proper medicines'. However, another man from Inchture was deemed unsuitable for admission as he 'only required sea bathing' which could be 'met by taking lodgings in town'. A long list of rules applied to patients, including that they were not to play at cards, dice, or any other games, not to smoke tobacco in the wards, not to throw any dirt or any other thing over the windows:

> Nursing was of the Sarah Gamp order, with little or no distinction between nurses and servants. Their conduct was often in question, although doubtless kind according to their lights, they had to be reminded that they must not neglect, insult or quarrel with the patients on any pretext whatever. Throughout the history of the old infirmary the illicit use of ardent spirits, sometimes introduced by means

of strings handed over the wall from the Bucklemakers' Wynd, continued to hamper the endeavours of the board to establish an efficient nursing service. The first nurse was appointed at 6s a week with board, joined later by a second day nurse, who received £12 a year, with board, but furnishing herself with tea and sugar.

The report notes it was the arrival of Strong which was to transform the service into one 'well in advance' of any other Scottish hospital of the time. Her appointment is noted in a newspaper report of 1 January of that year, which indicates that she had to battle some competition for the post:

> Mrs Rebecca Strong, late of the Royal Victoria Hospital, Netley, England, was yesterday elected matron of the Dundee Royal Infirmary, vacant by the removal of Miss Mercer to England. The election was unanimous. There were fourteen applicants for the situation.[2]

At a meeting of the governors of the hospital in March that year, it was clear there was great anticipation of what she would bring to the role. Her arrival at the hospital was described by the chairman as 'one of the most important duties we have had to perform in the interest of our infirmary':

> The appointment of Mrs Strong, from St Thomas' Hospital, London, and the Royal Netley Hospital, leads us to hope that in due time the Committee will not be

disappointed, for, being a thoroughly trained nurse, she is quite competent to train others to these onerous duties. But Gentlemen, Mrs Strong and the medical officers must receive due support and encouragement at your hands in carrying out these necessary changes in the nursing … Mrs Strong and Dr Sinclair have already made a beginning in this direction of improved nursing arrangements and training.[3]

In her own words, when Strong arrived at the hospital she found Sinclair to be a medical superintendent of 'very advanced views in regard to nursing':

He had succeeded in having an addition made to the hospital to give single bedrooms to the nursing staff, also a dining-room and a sitting-room. There was no definite teaching given to the nurses. I think we were both rather inclined to the idea that given an ordinarily intelligent woman of good principle, she could, by attendance at the bedside under the instruction of the medical man, educate herself. As nursing stood at that time she could acquire by those means all that was required of her. With the rapid advance of medicine and surgery, discovery after discovery being made, it did not suffice, but this came much later.[4]

The working relationship between the duo proved to be a successful one, and over the next few years they managed to raise the standards of nursing in the department to one that was 'exceptionally high for the time':

> His forward-looking policy helped her to crystallise her own views on the necessary preparation of a nurse, and that with the rapid advance of medical and surgical knowledge this should not just be limited to attendance at the bedside under the instruction of the medical personnel.[5]

However, while the training was far better than previously, it is important to note at this stage there were no formalised lectures or teaching:

> Nurse training was still the traditional method of learning by experience on the wards at the time, Mrs Strong believed that an average intelligent woman could learn all that was required of a nurse by working on the wards, under the instruction of a medical man.[6]

By the time Strong arrived, the hospital was very different from the early days of the apothecary and pigs. The average number of patients at any time was just 100–130; in 1879 the total for the year was 1,735, of whom 78 were under 10 and only 104 over 60:

> She was in charge of 18 nurses (of whom 6 were probationers) and 19 servants, plus porters and firemen.

In fact, the major part of her reforms seems to have been concerned with improving conditions. One of the first things she did was to put pictures on the walls of the wards. The directors provided help from a special fund to build new accommodation, pay was increased, working hours were reduced, and nurses were no longer required to do menial tasks. Probationers learned by being paired with qualified staff, and were given two hours' instruction a week from the Medical Superintendent.[7]

The annual report of the infirmary in 1875 – just a year after Strong's arrival – notes the progress which had been already made, with a £10,000 bequest used to fund the introduction of the 'training establishment of nursing':

[This] has raised the status of the nurses, and placed the nursing arrangements of the House upon an efficient and satisfactory basis. Adequate and suitably extended accommodation for carrying out this system having recently been completed, the services of several well-trained nurses and promising probationers have been secured, and the system is now fairly inaugurated under the direct superintendence of the Matron, who by her training is eminently qualified for this work, and very desirous of its success.[8]

These improvements were said to have resulted in raising standards to a high level within just a few years:

Nurses were remarked on for their 'exceptional neatness'
and the Directors noted 'the combined gentleness
and firmness ... characteristics of the Matron, who
treats the nurses and all the servants rather as sisters
or daughters engaged with her in a benevolent work
... studying their welfare and appealing to that self-
respect which establishes a high moral tone throughout
the whole service' and creates 'mutual good feeling and
confidence, and a happy cheerful spirit'.[9]

Strong was only connected to Dundee Royal Infirmary for
around five years, but in that time made a huge difference
to the standard of nursing care at the hospital. She was also
involved in other pioneering projects, such as the opening
of convalescent home next to the infirmary in 1876. This
was intended to be an 'intermediate place' between hospital
and discharge and was built with accommodation for fifty
patients. Strong was thanked at the opening for her assistance
in the furnishing of the home.[10]

A tradition of giving patients a Christmas party also
began while Strong was at Dundee Royal Infirmary, funded
by donations from supporters of the hospital. The first took
place in the year she joined the hospital and reports suggest
it was an occasion in which everyone became involved, with
Sinclair and Strong supervising the decorations.[11] It gives
an insight into the life at the hospital at the time Strong was
matron. One of the wards was set aside for the occasion and
as well as patients there were friends and supporters of the

infirmary attending. Around fifty of the ninety-two patients in the infirmary attended the entertainment, with around twenty patients who had been discharged in the previous week also invited to join in:

> The entrance hall and the corridor leading to the place of meeting were tastefully decorated with evergreens and illuminated balloons. The interior of the ward was also beautifully decorated with festoons of evergreens stretched across the rood, from which hung rows of illuminated balloons. All around the walls were displayed beautiful devices in evergreens and bannerets, interspersed with appropriate mottoes. But the most prominent object in the large hall was a lofty and spreading Christmas tree, lighted up with thousands of coloured tapers, and the branches loaded with valuable presents for all the patients and officials of the Institution. The decorations were designed by Mrs Strong, and executed by the nurses under her superintendence.[12]

Strong kept in touch with Dundee Royal Infirmary throughout her life and in 1929, at the age of 81, she revisited to open the Preliminary Training School for Nurses. A newspaper report of the time[13] notes that it was made possible through funding from James Prain, one of the directors, who donated the house at 5 Dudhope Terrace and provided the equipment. The school was named the Prain Preliminary Training School for Nurses and had accommodation for seven trainees. The description of their training shows just how far the education of nurses had developed since Strong was matron of the infirmary:

> Prior to entering upon their duties in the wards of the infirmary, these nurses for a period of two months will reside at the school, preliminary training being given by the sister in charge. They will receive instruction in elementary nursing and attend lectures on such subjects as ethics and the practice of nursing, hygiene, anatomy, and physiology. Thus at the termination of the training period they are better fitted to undertake the duties of the wards than if they entered these immediately. The change in environment, too, is more gradual and this is another advantage.

The report highlights other features of the new school – including bedrooms furnished in a 'bright and up-to-date manner', a cosy shared sitting room and a well-equipped lecture room:

> Mrs Strong opened the door of the school with a gold key, which Mr Prain handed to her and which bore the inscription 'Presented to Mrs Strong at the opening of the Prain Preliminary Training School for Nurses, 10th December, 1929'.

In her address, Rebecca said the experience of half a century was with her from the time she had held office there as matron. She outlined the events which led up to her being the instigator of the first nursing school in Glasgow, and spoke of the far-reaching benefits such a school as that she was opening would have:[14]

On first receiving Miss Niccol's letter I was elated with pleasure to think that the Infirmary in which I commenced work in a responsible position, had now arrived at a point in which it can claim to be one of the leading schools in Scotland for the study of nursing. Then I thought of those far distant days when both medicine and nursing were emerging from darkness into light. The days of Lister had so far advanced that we were enveloped in carbolic steam as an antiseptic at operations and the dressings that followed, but the day of aseptic work had scarcely dawned. This Infirmary when I had the honour of being appointed as Matron, was remarkably blessed in having a Medical Superintendent of the most advanced views, so much so that an addition was being built to give fitting accommodation to the nursing staff, some single bedrooms, and some double, a dining room, also a sitting room, a most unusual thing in those days, in fact scarcely thought of, so you see Dundee Royal Infirmary has never lacked enterprise. Previous to my being appointed Matron at the Dundee

Royal Infirmary, I spent 5 and half years in connection with the Nightingale School which was established at St Thomas' Hospital, London, where a custom was introduced, after I had joined the school, of having 'Lady Probationers' which induced some women of high position to enter, for which they paid, remaining one year as probationer, and then receiving the higher appointments. A school in the strict sense of the word it was not, no systematic teaching nothing but a stray lecture or two in the course of the year; it may be said it was empirical learning, each one making the best of her opportunities. There was a skeleton in a cupboard in our dormitory, and a few odd books on Anatomy of which some of us availed ourselves. We were very fortunate in having an excellent Resident Medical Officer who took great interest in us, and we were free to ask questions of him, and he of us, and thereby learnt a good deal.

Strong said that on being appointed matron at Dundee Royal Infirmary, she had 'no fixed ideals to aim at', other than being kind to patients, preventing bedsores and watching for changes in patients' health. But she said she had found an 'able, willing teacher' in Sinclair and that later work in developing nurse training at Glasgow Royal Infirmary had contributed to the opening of the Prain school:

The confidence of ignorance carried me through, and I spent a very happy and instructive time, to myself, in this Hospital, and on being appointed Matron to the Royal Infirmary, Glasgow, I found the experience gained here invaluable, but still no thought of systematic instruction for pupil nurses occurred to me, and when some classes were introduced to give a little technical teaching it was weary work for all, no time available, the whole time was required for bedside work, and not sufficient numbers to do that properly. However, we struggled on till a light seemed to dawn upon me that the whole business was unsatisfactory, and unless some big movement was made I would give it up, which I did, and opened a Home for Private patients in Glasgow, which kept me in touch with some of the medical men of Glasgow. When the position of Matron was again vacant, and I was asked to send in an application, I was better prepared to carry out the needs, and I was assured that the necessary support would be given. A system for the introduction of a preliminary course of instruction for pupil nurses had been drawn up by some of the Medical Staff of the Infirmary, and the consent of the Managers was easily gained. One of the results of that work is the opening of this School today.

The contribution Strong made to the infirmary was not forgotten and she attended staff reunions into her nineties. Long after she left, her ideas were influencing the matrons who succeeded her. A report noted that in 1939 a reunion of nurses at the hospital had sent greetings to the former matron, who by that time was 'within four years of being a centenarian':

> Mrs Strong attended the first reunion of DRI trained nurses three years ago, when she was the central figure of a company of about 160. About 10 years ago, she had the unique honour of opening the Prain School for preliminary training in nursing in Dudhope Terrace. This innovation was introduced by Miss Niccol, the present matron, who had, incidentally, trained under Mrs Strong in Glasgow, and who has been successful in putting into practice some of her teacher's ideas.[15]

On reaching her hundredth birthday in 1943, local papers in Dundee highlighted the city's connection with 'Britain's oldest nurse'. She also penned a letter to her well-wishers in Dundee which read:

> My dear friends, I am very grateful for your kind congratulations. My success has been owing to the strenuous efforts of those who worked with me. The advance is great since then and going on, you are blessed indeed with the good education in theory before being set to the practice of your Profession. Wishing you a long and happy life. Sincerely yours, Rebecca Strong.[16]

Strong's contribution to the city is marked on Dundee Women's Trail, which has a series of informative blue plaques throughout the city celebrating the achievements and contributions of twenty-five women who had a lasting impact. Her plaque can be found at Dunhope Park, opposite the gates of the former Dundee Royal Infirmary, which was finally closed in 1998 after 200 years of operation, to be replaced with the current Ninewells Hospital as the city's main hospital.

Chapter Four

A Turbulent Time at Glasgow Royal Infirmary

S trong had made her mark on Dundee Royal Infirmary, but the lure of moving to a bigger hospital meant that in 1879 she applied to Glasgow Royal Infirmary for the position of matron.

In her memoir, *Reminiscences*, Strong summed up her initial time at the Glasgow hospital saying when she was appointed she was 'not prepared for the backward condition of things':

> However, on the matter being placed before the Managers, they saw the necessity of moving on, and very quickly devised means for giving better arrangements all round for the nursing staff. I am afraid I was a rather troublesome woman, as soon as one step was taken I proposed another: this went on for a few years until it came to my asking for a 'Home' for the nurses, which was too much, and I was told quite plainly that I had gone too far, and, as I knew the work could not advance without it, I resigned, not wanting to see the work of the last few years lost.

This was in 1885. Her stint at Glasgow Royal Infirmary had come to an end just six years after her arrival. What led to the hospital board letting her go? Was she really such a 'troublesome woman' as she described herself?

When Strong arrived at Glasgow Royal Infirmary, the hospital was the largest voluntary hospital in Scotland with 579 beds. It had a nursing staff of sixty-two nurses and twenty-nine probationers. She was appointed with a salary of £120 per year.[1]

As for the city itself, it was undergoing a massive transformation as it became established as the 'second city of the Empire' by the end of the nineteenth century. Industry was booming, businessmen, industrialists and entrepreneurs were making fortunes, and thousands of workers were employed in factories and offices. But Glasgow's economic success came with a price – the grim toll on the population's health:

> The population included large numbers of poorly paid unskilled workers with little job security, and unemployment was often high. Despite the activities of the Improvement Trust in the city centre, slums such as those in Cowcaddens and around Glasgow Cross remained among the most overcrowded in the country, and the levels of social degradation to be found there shocked even the most hardened social commentators. Alcoholism, crime and the illnesses and diseases associated with overcrowding and undernourishment were rife in slum areas. With thousands of coal-burning industries, a fog of atmospheric pollution hung over the city, and this, too, took its toll on the health of the citizens.[2]

Diseases such as tuberculosis and bronchitis were commonly seen on the wards, while the victims of industrial accidents – both male and female – also often had to be admitted for treatment.

Before taking up the post of matron, Strong was allowed to look around the hospital, which enabled her to give feedback on what she thought of the conditions there. The managers were said to have listened 'sympathetically' to her views – which included highlighting a lack of domestic help on the wards, poor feeding arrangements and nurses having to sleep in 'nooks and crannies'.[3]

Nurses were divided into day and night nurses, assigned to one ward where they worked exclusively for one doctor or surgeon. However, there were some signs of attempting an improvement of standards – instead of relying on nurses to clean the wards, cleaners had been employed two years before Rebecca's arrival. There was also some kind of training in place:

Probationers' training consisted of two years' work on the wards where they worked as assistants, one in each ward and the more experienced were selected to cover for the regular nurses who were on leave or sick. They received £12 a year while training, £20 when qualified, rising by £2 a year until it reached £30. The year before Mrs Strong was appointed, lectures on medical and surgical nursing had been introduced by two members of the medical staff and this had proved so successful it was decided to continue the practice. These lectures were open to the public on payment.[4]

With a busy city hospital to deal with, and improvement of nurses training on the agenda, Strong already had much on her plate as the new matron. But there was another issue she encountered: the junior medical staff known as physicians' and surgeons' assistants. The residents, who were required to have obtained a relevant medical degree or diploma before joining the hospital, were not always respectful of the rules – which appears to have resulted in clashes with Strong as the matron in charge, who believed they were too inexperienced to have sole authority in the wards:

> They insisted they had the authority to deal with situations arising there, in the absence of their chiefs, and they resented the matron questioning their demands for the transfer of nurses when they, the residents, deemed assistance necessary.

The medical superintendent, Dr Moses Thomas, was jealous of his rights as the executive officer of the infirmary to countermand the matron's decisions, and she became convinced that he would always take the residents' side in any dispute which arose. Matters came to a head at Christmas 1881, apparently after the matron issued an instruction that the residents' dining room should close at an early hour in the evening, and the residents became openly rude and discourteous to her.[5]

The hostilities continued – so much so in that August 1882, Strong put in her resignation complaining of the conduct of the residents towards her as well as citing a difference in attitude towards the running of the hospital with the superintendent. In return, the superintendent defended himself by saying Strong was impatient and hasty, but was criticised in a report for defying her authority as the matron.

Strong delayed her resignation and won an important battle when the managers told her that in future she would be in sole charge of where the nurses were placed, subject to revision by the superintendent of the hospital:

> The matron had won a significant victory, establishing her authority over the junior doctors in nursing matters in the wards, and her right to communicate directly with the superintendent and visiting staff on matters relating to the nursing staff.[6]

Strong also had to deal with the demands of William Macewen, the eminent surgeon and pupil of Joseph Lister, who continued work in antiseptics and made revolutionary advances in the areas of bone, spinal cord and brain surgery. He had a major role to play in persuading Strong to join him at Glasgow Royal Infirmary and their relationship is explored further in this book. But particularly during this time, the relationship was not always an easy one.

Macewen was insistent that he needed probationer nurses to help with his pioneering surgical work, so that they could assist with observations. But when Strong agreed to his requests, it only served to irk other surgeons and their residents. A group of 'Macewen's nurses' became particularly loyal to the surgeon, so much so that they even clubbed together to buy him a fish kettle so he could sterilise his surgical instruments.[7]

And this fierce loyalty also meant that the nurses sometimes clashed with Strong. On one occasion in 1882, the matron complained to Macewen that a relief nurse had told her she took her orders from one of the surgeon's residents – not her. It was not the first time this had happened. Remembering the backdrop of her efforts in trying to transform the reputation of nurses, Strong was also distressed when the same resident – Dr David Potts – announced his engagement to one of the nurses. In a letter to Macewen, she outlined her concerns, saying that 'to govern ninety women under the most favourable circumstances is not an easy task' and the prospect of her nurses forming emotional attachments with the residents was not one to relish.[8]

In November 1882, Strong resigned from her position again, with the pressures of work having an impact on her mental health. However, ninety-two nurses signed a petition asking the managers to refuse to accept her resignation and she subsequently returned to work after doctors found she had recovered. After some turbulent years at Glasgow Royal Infirmary, Rebecca finally left in October 1885, explaining she was 'sorry my strength will not permit of my continuing so arduous and responsible a work for a long time'.

She also later spoke of her frustration at attempts to introduce some kind of class work for nurses saying, 'it was weary work; sleepy, tired nurses trying to take an interest in what they knew would be useful to them, and we unable to give them leisure.'[9]

She departed to open a private nursing home and later said her decision was prompted by the failure of the hospital board to build a new nurses' home, which she had been seeking since her arrival in Glasgow. This must have been a contrast to her experience in Dundee, where the new home was in place before her arrival – something which she believed was essential for the well-being of the nursing staff and vital for the aim of opening a school of nursing.

The managers in Glasgow had made some progress towards her request, including building a sitting room for off-duty nurses and converting an old dispensary into nineteen bedrooms for nurses. There were plans in place for a new nurses' home to accommodate thirty day nurses, twelve night nurses and ten probationers, but the managers had been unable to find an additional £5,000 of funding to build it by the time of Strong's departure from her post.

They were distressed to lose Mrs Strong, but they did finally authorise the building of the new home in the summer of 1886. It was opened on 31 August 1888, providing eighty-eight bedrooms. A glazed covered way (variously known over the years as 'the conservatory', 'the greenhouse corridor' and the 'hen run') was built to connect the home with the main buildings, offering shelter to nurses going to and from the wards, and exposing their visitors to the scrutiny of matron from her flat.[10]

After Strong left, a lady superintendent of nurses, Miss Wood, was appointed to take her place. But morale is said to have plummeted, with a new generation of younger women having greater expectations of the job and being less willing to tolerate the working conditions which older nurses had come to accept. Wood also found herself battling to improve conditions, with a request for the nursing staff to be increased by eight met with the response of managers placing a ward maid in each ward. In July 1891 she gave notice of her resignation.[11]

The troubles at the hospital continued. Later that year – six years after Strong left – the *North British Daily Mail* published an anonymous account of life as a nurse at Glasgow Royal Infirmary, under the name of 'a probationer'. The article claimed that while improvements were being made in many hospitals in England, this was 'by no means the case' at Glasgow Royal Infirmary:

It seems strange that an institution in which one would suppose health conditions would the supreme consideration we find the health of the workers systematically neglected and often wantonly sacrificed. This is all the more surprising when we remember that the Glasgow Royal Infirmary is one of the oldest, richest and most popular of institutions of its kind in the kingdom. Why it, then, should be behind others, here or elsewhere, in matters of 'improvement, progress or reform', is incomprehensible, not only to the nurses themselves, but also to members of the medical profession and the intelligent public who know anything of the management – or mismanagement! – of the nursing department in this infirmary.[12]

The scathing account of the conditions for nurses at the hospital continued, with the writer emphasising it was from her own experiences:

While all sorts and conditions of working-men are agitating for, and likely to obtain, a working day of eight hours, why should a day of fourteen and a half hours be exacted from the 'Royal' probationer nurse? She rises at 6 a.m. and continues 'on duty' until 8.30 p.m., with only half-an-hour for dinner, and a very uncertain interval of an hour and a half for rest or outdoor exercise. I say 'very uncertain' advisedly, for it is a deplorable fact that, on account of the scarcity of nurses, the probationer is too often obliged not only to sacrifice her precious hour and a half but also to remain 'on duty' till 10 p.m., in which case her day is one of sixteen hours.[13]

The probationer went on to highlight other examples of excessive working hours, stating she has previously worked 9 consecutive days on which she was regularly 'on duty' for 16 hours daily – equal to a 112-hour week. She also highlighted that probationers could be called at nights to do duties such as watching a patient in a side room or assisting in ward work from dawn until breakfast. In one case, a probationer – after complaining of completing a fourteen and a half hour day – was called at midnight to continue on duty until 5 p.m. the following day. She complained that there were no rules around holidays at Glasgow Royal Infirmary and that, during her year of probation, a nurse was also expected to attend lectures and classes and pass exams.

The food on offer to nurses in the dining room was also criticised – with potatoes 'rarely properly washed', a 'fearful and wonderful decoction called "stew"', and a milk pudding which is 'generally singed or otherwise rendered inedible'. The probationer concluded:

> Is it then surprising that the nurse of the 'Royal', devoted as she is to, and interested in her profession, does not consider her lot 'a happy one'? Several of the physicians and surgeons who have had a long connection with the institution have done much for

the nurses by expostulation with the authorities, and even by more practical measures, but although only a few of the difficulties of the nurse's life have been here mentioned, it will be seen that much yet remains to be done to make the 'Royal road' to learning nursing even moderately easy and attractive.

In conclusion, the writer would, in the name of the nurses of the Royal Infirmary, urge the Glasgow public, so famous for its ready sympathy and generosity, to inquire into the state of matters as above described; and, further, to see that justice, at least, shall be done to the nursing staff, whose lives are, essentially, full of noble purpose and self-sacrifice.

The account provoked a backlash, with the same paper the next day calling for the directors to publicly answer the 'grave statements' which had been made against the hospital, particularly over the length of the working day:

Such hours of work are monstrous. It is surely not necessary to kill the nurses in order to cure the patients. Such, however, would seem to be the system. But this raises another point, and it is one which concerns the public. If the nurses are kept on duty so long, can they give the patients all the attention which they ought to receive? We doubt it.[14]

The description of the food served to the probationer nurses also provoked criticism, while the management at the hospital were urged to speak out on what they would do to address the issues:

'All the food,' we are told, 'is miserably cooked and badly served.' If this be the case with regard to the food supplied to the nurses, is it the same with regard to the food supplied to the patients? On Sundays the nurses have invariably a cold dinner. Are the patients also restricted on Sundays to a cold dinner, without regard to their respective conditions, diseases, or injuries? If not, why are the nurses not as well treated as the patients? These are the questions which the directors must endeavour to answer to the satisfaction of the public. The indictment against the management of the Royal Infirmary is too serious to be met with silence. Indeed, this is one of those cases in which it would be held that 'silence gives consent'. The citizens of Glasgow have a right to know what defence, if any, can be offered. And they have a right, if the charges be true, to insist upon a reorganisation and reform of the management.

The controversy grew as more than seventy nurses supported the charges and the medical staff petitioned the hospital directors to hold an inquiry into the conditions for the nursing staff. *The Nursing Record* also took up the cause with editor

Mrs Bedford Fenwick even visiting Glasgow to investigate the claims – after which she concluded that the case has been 'understated rather than exaggerated':

> The facts stated, and which we have ourselves verified, prove that the arrangements in force at the Royal Infirmary are most inefficient. The first principle seems to be economy at any cost – not in anything else. The Managers, it would seem, have striven to show as large a number of patients, at as small an expenditure in pounds, shillings, and pence, as possible. Economy is most important, we admit, but we maintain that economy at the expense of efficiency, when life and death are concerned, is the most ridiculously wasteful policy possible. But the Managers of the Royal Infirmary – doubtless well-meaning, excellent gentlemen as individuals – are, as a Committee, clearly imbued with the crass idea that the success of a Hospital is show in its balance-sheet.[15]

The reports said the sanitary arrangements, especially with regard to 'lavatory accommodation', could 'not be believed except they were seen' and are a 'striking exemplification of the absolute carelessness of the health of the Nurses which exists at the Royal Infirmary, Glasgow'.

The hospital bosses attempted to downplay the criticism, as noted in *The Nursing Record*[16] which described a letter written to the *Daily Mail* by Mr William McEwen, who was appointed as a director of Glasgow Royal Infirmary in

1862, as something that would have 'overwhelmed the satirist who declared that Scotchmen have no sense of humour'. According to the report, he outlined how nurses at the time when he joined did not get a regular dinner but got 'a herring one day, a bit of cheese another, an egg upon the third, and picked up on other days anything that was to be had' and that the nurses slept in wards or in a row above the kitchen, and had to scrub floors. *The Nursing Record* scathingly noted: 'Mr McEwen gives Glasgow to understand that all this was altered for the better under his management.'

Fenwick made a series of recommendations to improve the nursing department, including the appointment of a nursing committee to oversee the department and to which a nurse could make a direct complaint, improving the nurses' diet, a minimum of two nurses on duty at every ward and three weeks' holiday each year for nurses and probationers. A subcommittee appointed to investigate the complaints published a report exonerating the managers from any blame, after an inquiry which interviewed twenty-three nurses:

The report listed the improvements which had been made in the nurses' conditions over the last 20 years, it stated that the food was adequate, the hours of work not unreasonable and the ratio of one nurse to five beds as good as in other hospitals.

The report did recommend an improvement in the nurses' holidays, increasing them to a month's leave, with at least 14 days in the summer. The appointment of a nursing committee to supervise the nursing department was also approved.[17]

Despite the managers downplaying the situation, the bid to highlight the unhappiness of the nurses with their working conditions at Glasgow Royal Infirmary had been successful, attracting interest from beyond the city. When it came to the appointment of a new matron, there was one candidate who was seen to be ideal for the job.

Chapter Five

'Setting Things Straight' in Glasgow

After Strong left Glasgow Royal Infirmary, she set up a small private nursing home in Glasgow. She ran the home for six years and said it helped to keep her in touch with nursing. She also kept in touch with Sir William Macewen during this time, with many of his private patients coming under her supervision.[1] Despite being away from the wards, the idea of improving training for nursing staff never left her, as she notes in *Reminiscences*:

During that time I was more and more impressed with the necessity for a definite education for the nurse if she was to meet the great advance that was being made both in medicine and surgery, being often at a loss myself, after my long experience, to fully understand the instructions given, but did not hesitate to ask for explanation when necessary, which was freely given. During those years I had many opportunities of taking over a curriculum for a nurses' elementary course of instruction, little thinking it would be my happy lot to have anything to do with carrying out of it.[2]

Meanwhile, the managers of Glasgow Royal Infirmary, no doubt keen to put the troubles of the nursing department behind them, appear to have 'headhunted' Strong for the position of matron again. Even though she had not had an entirely positive experience of working there the first time around, the offer of being able to develop her ideas on educating nurses was too tempting.

The Nursing Record reported that the directors had requested she return to the 'much-troubled institution' in order to 'set things straight' – and welcomed her appointment:

> This will be good news for the Nurses, as during her term of office she gained the respect and affection of her subordinates, as their well-being was always her first consideration. Mrs Strong is a lady of exceptional abil-ity, and practically returns to the Royal as a Dictator as it is only upon the promise of drastic reforms being inau-gurated in the Nursing Department that she consents to return at all. It will be remembered that she resigned from her post five years ago, owing to the constant fric-tion arising from the autocracy of a fellow official; but we should imagine that after the late expose and consequent indignation of the subscribers to the Institution, that she will not have to complain of this trouble for the future.[3]

However, the report also criticised the hospital at that time as being 'very much under-nursed'. It pointed out there were no sisters or head nurses, as in English hospitals, and the staff for a ward of twenty beds consisted of just one staff nurse, a probationer for day duty and a probationer for night duty:

> The Staff Nurse is usually an experienced woman; but when she is off duty the Ward, sometimes containing *twenty critical cases* is left in the entire charge of a Probationer of one day's experience and upwards. Probationers of six- or eight months' experience are placed in entire charge in the night and keep on permanent night duty for *two years or so*. The only chance these Probationers have of gaining practical experience is by remaining on duty until the mid-day. Such a system seems almost incredible in the latter half of the nineteenth century. The patients will never receive the skilled attention they require until the Nursing Staff is largely increased.[4]

Instead, it was stated, the ward should be staffed by one sister, one staff nurse and two probationers – with one staff nurse and one probationer on night duty:

> For a Ward containing more than twenty beds, a permanent Staff Day Nurse will be necessary, who shall be on duty at all times when the Sister is off duty. Considering the great wealth of the Glasgow Royal Infirmary, these reforms should be inaugurated at once.[5]

Strong's decision to go back to Glasgow Royal Infirmary is also thought to have been influenced and encouraged by the eminent surgeon Macewen, who was calling for improvements in the training of nursing. She alluded to this in her own recollections:

> In 1892 the office of Matron of the Royal Infirmary of Glasgow was vacant, and I had the honour of being asked to apply, which I did, and was appointed, and then began the happiest time of my life, everybody helpful and enthusiastic, and a home for the nurses was then in existence. The path of progress had been pointed out by the late Sir William Macewen, who, on the morning of 1st January 1891, in addressing the nursing staff, asked why should not nursing become a profession with its teachers, its examiners and its diploma?[6]

This referred to a key address given by Macewen, delivered in Glasgow Royal Infirmary, in which he set out his vision for the future of nursing. He praised the nurses he had worked with and said he had received from them 'such an amount of valuable hours of difficulty and trouble':

> In my practice, the assistant surgeons, the nurses, and myself, all pull in the same boat, with steady even strokes. We are actuated by the same aims and aspirations; they expect me to give them the latitude and longitude, and set them the course which I know

they will then steadily pursue. Every new operation advanced by me has been followed by the nurses with keen and discerning interest; and the success of many of these is in no small measure attributable to the care and attention which the nurses have devoted to them.

He described the nursing of the past as looming through the distance like a 'hideous nightmare', but that over the past decade a 'revolution' in nursing at Glasgow Royal Infirmary had been achieved, thanks to the contributions of figures such as Strong. However, he also warned that nursing was not yet in a 'satisfactory condition':

Though the few may be nearly perfect, the mass remains an untutored host, and unless possessed of extra individual energy, nurses simply float medusa-like through the wards into the stream of life – and we fold our hands and see them go! As they mingle in the street, the public cannot discern the spurious from the genuine article.

Cannot nursing be raised to a distinct profession, with its entrance examination, its minimum requirements, theoretical and practical, its teachers, its examiners and its diploma? Cannot St Mungo's College, with its omnivorous capacity, found a Faculty of Nursing? The whole machinery and material is at hand, the students are assembled, and are anxious and eager to begin.

Macewen set out the vision of a nurse acquiring knowledge in fields including anatomy, physiology, bacteriology, hygiene, cuisine and learning the principles of medicine and surgery, sufficient so that she can 'follow with intelligence the movements of disease, and the treatment she is entrusted to carry out'. He argued this training should be completed before she is allowed to have full charge of a ward and pupils should sit examinations to become 'Diplomates of Nursing of the Royal Infirmary'.

Macewen also emphasised the benefits for woman in having training for a profession so that they could be self-supporting:

The public would then have a guarantee that in employing such a nurse, they were receiving one thoroughly qualified. Will the Royal Infirmary lead in this direction, or will it wait till others take the field? Of course, nurses of this stamp would not engage in menial work, and I think all nurses ought to be relieved from such. Every girl, whatever her station in life may be, ought to be trained not only to be a useful member of society, but to be self-supporting. She ought to be taught a profession, an occupation, or a trade, whereby she could earn her own livelihood. Were this the case, the world would be the happier. An unmarried woman, who quietly and perseveringly makes her own way through life, unsupported by others and who retains her womanly characteristics, is worthy of the highest respect.

Of course, this was the late nineteenth century and so the views on the role of women often only extended so far – with Macewen arguing nursing was 'woman's work' and could not be done by a man as his 'instincts and training do not suit him for it':

> A woman is a born nurse. If one wishes to know the sex of a child, present it with a doll; and while a boy may look at is askance, take hold of it as he would a crab, or grasp it by the head or legs, and tuck it under his arm, a girl will crow with delight, seize it eagerly but tenderly and fold it to her breast, with many demonstrations of affection. The whole training of women fosters nursing. Man is more or less dependent upon women from his cradle to his grave.

However, that attitude was not shared by everyone and there was high demand for suitably trained men to care for male patients. The first nursing register contained the names of 24 men by the end of 1922, although that was in comparison to nearly 10,000 female nurses registered.[7] It is interesting to note that nursing is still one of the most gender-segregated jobs in the UK, with recent figures from the Nursing and Midwifery Council showing men made up just over 11 per cent of the registered nurses in the UK.[8]

Macewen also argued that religion should be the 'foundation from which nursing springs':

Those who feel that religion is not confined to forms, ceremonies, and repetitions of words, but that is consists of living acts inspired by the proper motive, will find in nursing an ennobling and truly religious work. To fan the flickering spark of life, to cheer the sufferer's couch, to soothe when earthly hope is fled, to soften the pillow of the dying, to dry the mourner's tears and to do these with self-abnegation, devotion to others, and patient endurance, is to live one's religion. It has been well said, 'It is better to make one's life a poem than to write one' and I would add, that the nurse who does her duty in the true spirit makes her life a prayer.

The return of Strong to Glasgow Royal Infirmary was of great significance – as someone known for battling to improve the conditions for nurses, it sent a signal that the hospital management was behind her vision:

Macewen was also reunited with the woman with whom he had collaborated on earlier innovations in nurses' education, and with whom he could work on the latest proposal – 'an establishment for a systematic course of training for nurses to be followed by examinations' – which he first suggested to the managers in April 1892, and which he presented in depth in October, only a few days before he resigned to become Regius Professor of Surgery at the University of Glasgow and a visiting surgeon at the Western.[9]

By the time Strong had returned to Glasgow Royal Infirmary, the new nurses' home had been built. However, there was a still an issue with understaffing of the wards, as had been noted in the account in the *Nursing Times*. The managers approved plans to build an additional storey to the nurses' home, which, once ready, enabled the nursing staff to be increased thanks to the provision of another twenty-two bedrooms:

> Mrs Strong was able to assign four nurses to each ward and to rearrange the hours of duty so that continuous night duty was abolished and replaced by a rotation of three months.[10]

When Strong had been matron previously, a series of lectures had been given to the nurse probationers, but this was deemed to interfere too much with the working of the wards and taking them away at irregular hours to attend the talks. Another issue was the nurses were not given any significant time to study away from the wards – which meant the lectures had limited usefulness as it was difficult for the probationers to undertake further study.

It was not long before Strong and Macewen proposed a major shake-up of the nurses' training – it was time to put their long-held ideas of reform into practice.

Chapter Six

The 'Art of Nursing' Begins

In April 1892, Macewen put plans for improving nurse training at Glasgow Royal Infirmary to the house committee and following a meeting with the medical committee, the details were decided upon. The new system began with the commencement of lectures on 10 January 1893 and it was to put the hospital at the forefront in the UK in the provision of preliminary training schools for nurses.

There were initial qualifications for entry: candidates had to either have obtained a Leaving Certificate of the Scottish Education Department or take an entrance exam, tested on grammar, spelling and arithmetic. The initial training lasted around three months and comprised two courses lasting six weeks each. The first covered lectures and demonstrations in anatomy, physiology and hygiene and were conducted by a professional. Each pupil paid a fee of 2 guineas for the course and also had to find her own board and lodging. Lectures were delivered on Tuesday and Thursday evenings at 7 p.m.

After successful completion of this initial course – which included passing an exam and the awarding of a certificate – the candidates went on to further clinical study in the form of lectures given both in the medical school at St Mungo's College and in Glasgow Royal Infirmary and demonstrations on surgical and medical cases, ward work and cookery – with the latter given by Strong herself. The fee for this course was 3 guineas and it lasted four weeks.

Passing this second course meant the candidates were now admitted as probationers – and could gain experience on the wards. This was two years' training, during which they received a wage of £12 in the first year and £20 in the second year, as well as free board and lodging. Once this training was completed, the final hurdle to gaining certification as a fully trained nurse was a written and practical exam.

The introduction of such a structured scheme of training and instruction – including before potential nurses got anywhere near the ward – was a radical change from what had gone before:

> The scheme was a new departure in nurse education in several ways. It pioneered the block system by dividing the nurses' training into blocks of lecture, followed by blocks of practical ward work. It introduced the idea of compulsory theoretical instruction and examination before probationers entered the wards, and inaugurated a systematic theoretical instruction in nursing. It set an educational standard for entry to the training, and initiated the practice that nurses should pay fees for their instruction.

> Most innovatively, it placed nurses' education in the medical college, making nurses potential students.[1]

When the prospectus was published, certain aspects of the scheme were criticised by nursing commentators – particularly the length of training and the amount of clinical instruction.

These concerns were outlined in an editorial in *The Nursing Record* devoted to discussing its introduction in January 1893. It noted that the introduction of the course reflected a prediction which the journal had made in 1889 that there would be a preliminary examination for nurses introduced for admission to a training school. It congratulated Strong and the Glasgow Royal Infirmary for initiating a system which 'we believe as firmly today, as we believed four years ago, will, with some differences of detail, become, in time, the recognised and general course of Nursing education.'[2]

However, it outlined in detail the two faults which it believed the scheme had – arguing the two years' practical ward training was too short and the six weeks' clinical instruction was too limited and given at a time when it would not be most useful to pupils:

The prospectus clearly provides that candidates, who have satisfied the Managers of their general educational acquirements, and who have successfully proved their knowledge of the subjects taught to them in the Lectures on Anatomy, Physiology, and Hygiene, must, before they enter the Wards as Probationers, furthermore attend a course of lectures and demonstrations on medical cases, surgical cases, ward work, and cookery. Now, this appears to us, for various reasons, to be a mistake. Turning, for a moment, to the education of medical students, we find that they are compelled to spend the first eighteen months or so of their curriculum in the study, at the College attached to the Hospital, of theoretical subjects. Their knowledge of these subjects is then tested by examination, and if they are found proficient, then, and not until then, they commence their work in the Wards. Concurrently with, and explanatory of, the actual cases which they see, they receive clinical instruction. But, in the case of Nurses – who have not had, and cannot of course, obtain, the complete knowledge of the human organism in health, which prepares the medical student to understand the effects produced upon it various accidents and diseases – it is, surely, somewhat premature to give lectures and demonstrations upon surgical and medical cases concerning whose past history these ladies will know but little, and whose future progress they will probably comprehend still less.

The editorial argued this theoretical instruction would be quickly forgotten because the pupils would not have the chance to put it into practice immediately. It suggested some changes – such as having housekeeping part of the preliminary education exam and including the course on cookery in the first course.

Despite these concerns, the training programme was a huge success in terms of attracting applicants. Just one advert was needed to fill the first class with a high quality of candidates and this never had to be repeated – as outlined in a letter written by Strong nearly fifty years later:

> So popular did it become, one advertisement sufficed to carry through the 16 years (my second period of office as Matron) … unnecessary to say it attracted a fine type of womanhood.[3]

Some years after it was set up, Strong described her reaction to seeing her ambition for a nursing school finally realised, in an interview: 'The relief was immense, and we all began to enjoy our work, relieved of the incubus of mixing study with it.'[4]

In November 1894, two years after the scheme was introduced, Strong was invited to give a paper to the first meeting of the Matrons' Council in London. She was pleased with the results of the training initiative, but only one or two hospitals had taken it up and it was to be a number of years before it would become widespread. The emphasis of the talk, therefore, was that nurses' education was still very much in its infancy – which is not surprising, given that when it was made the first candidates at Glasgow Royal Infirmary had not yet completed their two years' probation in the wards or sat their final exam.

In the 'Education in Nursing' speech, Strong said the early stages of a system so recently inaugurated must be 'largely tentative until tested by practical experience'. But she noted:

We have made a departure from the old paths, whether better remains to be proved. We do not depreciate the work of the past; it served its time; and without the labours of our predecessors we should not stand where we are today. Life should be growth or progress. Let us endeavour to add something to the stores of the past that may help forward the work of the future. To make our position clear we must take a cursory glance over the field of nursing – past and present.

She highlighted the 'impetus given to nursing' given by her mentor Florence Nightingale and subsequent establishment of her training school in conjunction with Wardroper, whom Miss Nightingale 'found quietly working in St Thomas's Hospital, seeking to rescue during from its degraded position'. Strong said the best way to pay tribute to 'these noble women' was to expand on the work which they had begun. She said that if the training school at St Thomas' Hospital remained the only one in the UK there would have been a uniformity of education and argued it could have met the demands of better qualifications for the nursing. But she noted:

As it is, almost every hospital in the kingdom followed the laudable example set by the 'Nightingale Committee' and instituted 'Training Schools' each being a law unto themselves. Hence the great variety in the forms of 'education' introduced, which has called forth the desire for uniformity, both in instruction and in the test to be applied before 'Diplomas in Nursing' are granted. As nursing stands now, it has no definite position. There is no uniformity of education, no general test or examination to prove whether a woman is qualified to take charge of the sick or not.

Strong said this made nursing certificates 'comparatively speaking, worthless' unless someone had an intimate knowledge of each hospital and knew exactly how the certificate had been achieved. She also pointed out that some still believed that twelve months spent in a hospital without any theoretical instruction would be enough for a woman to pick up sufficient knowledge to be able to undertake the duties of a nurse:

This implies that a nurse's work is purely mechanical, requiring little mental capacity. In days gone by, when the whole treatment of the sick was of a different nature – a nurse's work consisting largely of giving medicines at certain intervals, gratifying the patient's wishes as much as possible, no scientific report being required of the patient's varying changes and symptoms – the so-called 'training' was sufficient. I trust the custom is now obsolete of 'ladies' going into hospital, paying a considerable sum, remaining only one year, then receiving or obtaining appointments of considerable importance and assuming the title of 'trained nurse'.

Strong said knowledge gained at the bedside over years by a 'fairly intelligent woman' could produce a 'most valuable nurse' – but that this had to go alongside considering the number of failures 'partly owing to the want of a natural ability for observation' and 'partly owing to the want of direct instruction'. Advances in medicines brought with it the need for a 'systematically instructed nurse', who should have knowledge of a 'definite nature', she argued:

> Given a 'trained nurse', there should be some standard or test, so that anyone employing her many have some idea of what to expect from her. Degrees of knowledge will ever be regulated by the power of the individual to assimilate the instruction given; still there should be a fixed quantity.

She said some hospitals had introduced lectures for their probationers, which had to be attended alongside gaining experience of work, but warned that this system – which had been previously the custom at Glasgow Royal Infirmary – 'seriously interfered' with the work of the wards, including having probationers taken away at irregular hours for attending lectures. Another issue she pointed out was that the trainee nurses could not be given any time for study outwith attending the lectures – which rendered them 'practically useless for the majority' who could not fit it in during their rest time:

This led to the consideration of a long-projected scheme, viz, the taking of a special course of instruction including Elementary Anatomy, Physiology, and Hygiene, followed by a course of Clinical instruction, before being admitted into the wards for the learning of the practical part of a nurse's work, By the aid of our medical staff this matter was placed before our managers, and received by them with the most hearty sympathy. After due consideration a scheme was elaborated which we were requested to put into operation in January 1893. As far as we can judge it appears to be a success.

Strong acknowledged there were initial difficulties but said they were 'no means formidable' and that medical staff had cooperated 'most heartily' to facilitate the idea – and said that the hospital was already benefiting from having better-trained nurses. She outlined how class certificates were given at the end of each course of lectures, stating the percentage of marks received by each pupil for exams in the different subjects. But she said there was not yet an arrangement for a final examination before granting diplomas, hoping that 'this may be taken out of our hands by an independent body of examiners in connection with registration':

If the Royal British Nursing Association [RBNA] could see its way to establishing such a Committee, representing England, Scotland, and Ireland, to examine and decide a nurse's qualifications before she is placed on their Register, it would give prestige to those nurses. This appears a formidable suggestion, but if deliberately considered I think it may assume a practicable form. There would be expense connected with it, as the examiners must have their fees. The examination fees to be paid by nurses would defray this expense; but what would be of more serious consideration would be the arranging of the examining centres for the three countries, as the nurses would have to go to the examiner, and they could scarcely be asked to congregate in London. If centres could be established in the three countries, it would make it comparatively easy for nurses to present themselves.

Strong said for the RBNA to step forward and take steps to introduce a fixed curriculum with a diploma qualification for women wishing to become nurses would not generate 'more opposition that it has done in the past' and would gain supporters. She envisaged that the association might be to the nursing world what the General Medical Council – which had been established in 1858 – was to the medical world. She said at present the RBNA did not meet requirements and should ensure the full qualification of a woman for nursing, rather than the current arrangements which means it accepts the certificate of any hospital containing a certain number of beds, which certifies the nurse to have been resident for not less than three years but without any special test to ascertain the status of the nurse:

I repeat, mere residence in a hospital will not qualify. The authorities of hospitals do not pay a uniform attention to the training of their nurses. Some women during the period of their probation, to a large extent, educate themselves; others again wait for a teacher. Many people say education will not make a nurse. The point is, can they be made without it? Is it the solitary profession that requires no special instruction? Will instinct supply all that is necessary to meet they myriad wants of the sick? I think not.

Strong said after nearly thirty years' experience of being a nurse and dealing with nurses, she was impressed with the idea that, 'we are only just beginning to realise what the art of nursing may become if proper means are used for its development.' She said she thought it would become one of the best openings for women who will 'apply themselves to acquiring the knowledge' – and while it would involve some expense for individuals, this was only in common with other forms of employment:

> Nursing can demand remuneration on an average with other livelihoods or women, and why the preliminary cost it entails for special instruction should be looked upon as a hardship any more than special instruction for other purposes, I do not know.

Strong said nurses under the old regime were appreciative of the advances in training and largely making themselves available for instruction, while medical staff were also encouraging. She said it was to them they looked for assistance in the further development of the scheme and better regulation of nurses:

> It has been remarked to me that that, in seeking to obtain a 'standard of education' for women wishing to qualify as nurses, we are losing sight of the morale or character of the nurse, and seeking only professional skill. In the event of legislation being obtained there would be a Register published annually, stating a nurse's qualifications: and in the event of her committing any flagrant act against the recognised code of morals, her name would be struck off the Register. Others again suggest that a State regulation of a nurses' curriculum would interfere with the power exercised over the 'nursing staff' by hospital authorities. I cannot see how this can be. All that the Crown would do would be to regulate the instruction given and the class certificates to be held before entering the wards of a hospital, the time spent in hospital also to be fixed by the State. During the time spent in the wards she would be fully under the control of the hospital authorities, and would in no way interfere with the discipline of these institutions.

Strong also argued that nurses who wanted to specialise in particular areas should undergo the general training, before going on to further study – arguing that having a wider background of 'illnesses of all kinds' would help deal with unexpected situations. But she noted the current facilities for special purposes were limited. She also said it would be necessary to take into account those nurses who were already working:

> In the event of a compulsory form of education being introduced, with its examination and diploma, it would be necessary to consider the position of those nurses already in practice. Probably this might be met by placing them on the Register with some distinctive qualification indicating the degree of qualification. 'Graduate in Nursing' appears a fitting title for one fully qualified to practise the art.

Strong concluded by saying her remarks were 'crude' and called for further discussion and debate on the issue:

> It is by this means we can gather up the different aspects of the question. No two people take exactly the same view of things.

The paper was published in the *Nursing Record* in November 1894 and was discussed at a meeting that same month – believed to be the first time matrons had met together as hospital officials to discuss their work and duties.[5] The Matrons' Council had only just been set up, with Strong appointed as vice chairman.[6]

Strong's proposals were described as 'admirable', but concern was raised about the cost of such a scheme – with the argument that although this might not be excessive in Glasgow, it would be in a place like London. One doctor's remarks were reported:

> He believed that many who enter the career of Nursing have practically no means; and he feared that to impose an entrance fee in the shape of an expensive preliminary education would tend to deprive many who would make excellent Nurses of the power to enter the profession. However, he hoped the paper would circulated, and be read not only by Nurses, but by Hospital Managers and the general public.

Another attendee pointed out that men wishing to train as doctors also potentially faced a similar issue:

> She supposed the expense of becoming a doctor was a bar to many promising young men; and many would like to go to the Universities but could not afford it. But it has never been suggested that medical or University fees should in consequence be done away with ... Of course some women would be prevented from becoming Nurses because of the initial fees; but the standard should not be lowered to save a few poor women.

In response to the various concerns raised, Strong said the curriculum drawn up by teachers at Glasgow Royal Infirmary was not being promoted with the idea that it would form a model for other schools – although that is what eventually happened. She also said it was hoped that bursaries and grants would be awarded in the future to help those who would otherwise be unable to meet the costs of training.

Strong's paper was also published in an American journal, *The Trained Nurse*, a year later, under the title 'Education in Nursing'. While Strong had been keen to emphasise the training course was only in the early stages, it quickly became a model for nursing schools in America, where nurse education was developing rapidly:

> The article was published in the influential American Journal of Nursing in February 1901, and in the following issue, Adelaide Nutting, Superintendent of Nurses at the Johns Hopkins Hospital, Baltimore, and one of the leaders in the development of nurse education, paid tribute to the lead which the Glasgow Royal Infirmary had given to schools of nursing in all countries. In her article, Miss Nutting pointed out that the development of a systematic course of theoretical instructions for nurses brought nursing into line with all other branches of education, whether in art, trade or the professions.[7]

In 1901, Strong had appeared on the programme of the International Nurses' Congress in Buffalo, New York, to give a talk on the subject of 'The Preparatory Instruction of Nurses'.[8] However, she was unable to attend after being taken ill in Philadelphia.[9] The development of the course at Johns Hopkins was subsequently described in detail during a meeting of The International Congress of Nurses in 1902:

> I was at the Johns Hopkins some time ago and saw the beginning of the six months' course. The six months' preparatory course is in reality a part of the three years' course. The whole of the Nurses' Home has been turned into what you might call a laboratory; a working laboratory. During this six months the pupils do not go into the wards. The junior class, half of them coming in the spring, and half in the autumn, go at once into this preparatory school. While they are there they are taught every branch of domestic training. They are taken out to market, and are taught to inspect foods, supplies, and to purchase in small and large quantities; in wholesale and retail; to arrange different kinds of food, etc. Then they enter the kitchen and prepare all the food for the whole training school. When I was there they were already preparing the breakfasts and suppers for the whole training school of seventy-five pupils.

The trainee nurses spent a certain time in the kitchen, where they also learned to prepare 'dainty dishes' for individual patients. Another area of learning was in practical housework from the 'work of the kitchenmaid to that of the chambermaid', so that they know how to 'direct servants' and the time taken to complete particular tasks:

> They thoroughly do every kind of work in and about the hospital so they will never be embarrassed when confronted by questions of that kind when taking hospitals in charge themselves. They do not keep on doing one kind of work, but pass through each department, and the coming nurses take their places. Their bedrooms are in the most beautiful order. West Point does not come up to them; they are perfect. During this six months they also study their hygiene, anatomy, and physiology. They have also practical demonstrations in the elementary part of the nurse's work. They learn to make dressings and the surgical supplies and appliances they have in the wards, consequently when they go into the wards I think you must agree that they start with much more confidence and do very much better work. It is a very expensive course, and requires quite a staff of teachers, and altogether very few hospitals could ever establish such a course. But the Johns Hopkins School serves as an object lesson and in time we might have central schools in all cities where all probationers may be received before going into the hospitals.

Strong also continued to make improvements to conditions at Glasgow Royal Infirmary, where a steady rise in the number of patients was resulting in a demand for new departments. When the managers drew up plans for a rebuilding programme in 1899, she was asked to outline the requirements for the nursing and domestic staff. The nursing staff had increased to 134 and with the hospital accommodation full, various lodgings in the neighbourhood were also being used to house them. So the new building programme included a home which had space for ninety nurses and included sitting rooms, a dining room, kitchen, sick room, a servants' house and apartments for matrons and housekeepers.

Strong was also instrumental in ensuring that nurses received better pay and conditions; in that same year, she recommended changes to help ensure that the trained nurses remained at the hospital and were not tempted to move elsewhere. This included having the maximum salary of £30 per year reached after five years instead of seven and in 1901, the top pay was increased to £35.[10]

The success of her training scheme resulted in demand for nurses trained at Glasgow Royal Infirmary; in 1898, the annual meeting of the hospital board noted comments from Strong that they had recently lost some of their best nurses, with four going to South America and two going to South Africa. Strong said this was regrettable – but also that the hospital was proud of their achievements.[11]

Strong's second period as matron lasted sixteen years until 1907, when she was aged 64 and retired after being granted three months leave on health grounds. When she gave notice of her intention to leave, she said she found the work too fatiguing and could not face another winter. But before she left in August, she attended the laying of the memorial stone for the new buildings which she had helped to plan – an elaborate occasion which was attended by around 4,000 people:

> The ceremony of laying the memorial stone of the new and reconstructed buildings of Glasgow Royal Infirmary by His Royal Highness the Prince of Wales was carried through in the most brilliant fashion. The sun shone brightly on a scene notable for its gaiety and variety, and although the wind occasionally blew half a gale, it caused little or no discomfort. Preparations on an elaborate scale had been made by the managers of the Infirmary for the ceremonial of the day. The great square of the institution had been transformed into an amphitheatre, which gave accommodation for about four thousand spectators. In the centre was a high raised platform, over the middle of which swing the memorial stone in readiness to be lowered into its place. The platform was roofed over with crimson and white cloth: the supporting pillars were wreathed in tartan of the Stewart and Rothesay pattern: and lordly deers' heads, in antlered glory, were conspicuous ornaments.[12]

Strong's time at Glasgow Royal Infirmary had come to an end. Her legacy was a transformation in the training of nurses at the hospital which provided inspiration around the world.

Chapter Seven

Campaigning for Registration and a New Club for Nurses

S trong may have retired from Glasgow Royal Infirmary but her work with the nursing profession was far from over. As well as receiving a pension of £120 per year from the hospital, she was also left a legacy of £6,000 in 1908 by Dr David McCowan of Glasgow, who was impressed by her work during the time she was matron at the hospital. He was a chief partner in the firm of Messrs William Euing and Co and left large bequests to employees, servants and public and charitable institutions, including £5,000 to Glasgow Royal Infirmary.[1]

A major area of work where she continued after her retirement was the issue of state registration for nurses, of which she was a supporter. This was an idea that had first been proposed by the president of the General Medical Council Dr Henry Acland, in 1874. But it was to be many years before such a system came into being, when the passing of the Nurses' Registration Act in 1919 led to the setting up of the General Nursing Council. In between, there were debates over what the register should look like – including whether it should actually be compulsory and if a single register should be set up across Britain.

In 1887, the British Nurses' Association was set up and two years later it passed a resolution calling for the opening of a register. It later received a royal charter in 1892 to become the Royal British Nurses' Association (RBNA).

A report from a meeting of the Association for Promoting the State Registration of Nurses summarised the debate over why a formal system was needed from various voices:

> [The Marchioness of Londonderry] said the public had a right to know if the nurse they employed had a thorough training. Women who had only a few months' training could now compete with those who had spent four or more years in qualifying, and could demand the same pay. Miss Isla Stewart, matron of St Bartholomew's Hospital, remarked that although nursing was the most important of professions for women, the management of the profession was not in the hands of nurses. There was no standard of proficiency. Miss Mollett, matron of the Royal South Hants and Southampton Hospital, spoke strongly in favour of registration. No one, she said, wanted to do away with trained nurses. It was a free country, and any who wished to employ them could do so: but it was the 'mock nurses' who were objected to – women who dressed in nurses' uniform and took the pay for qualified nurses, and against who the public were not now protected.[2]

In 1905, a House of Commons select committee was set up to examine the issue of nurse registration and concluded

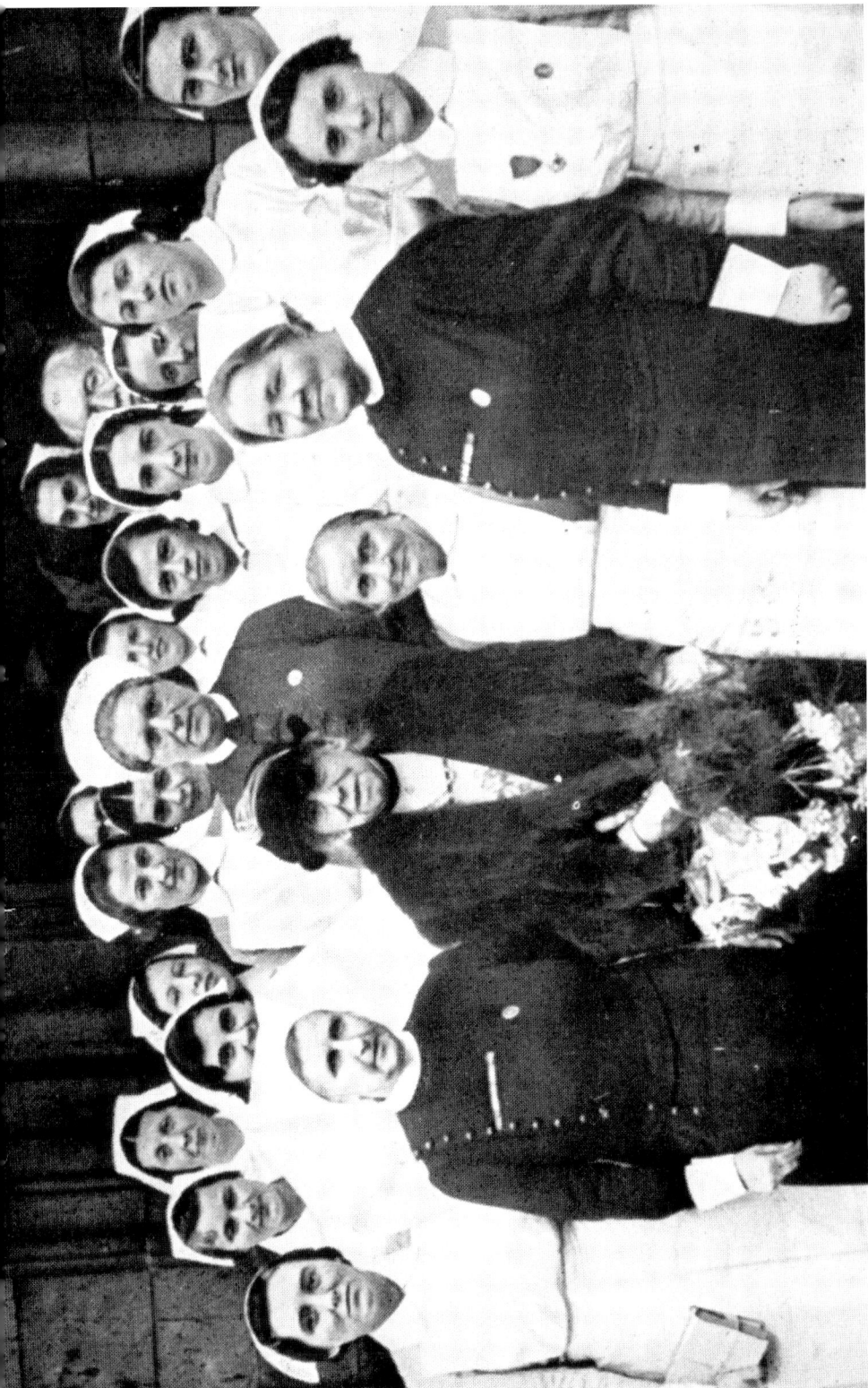

Rebecca Strong with group of nurses, Glasgow Royal Infirmary. (Courtesy of NHS Greater Glasgow and Clyde)

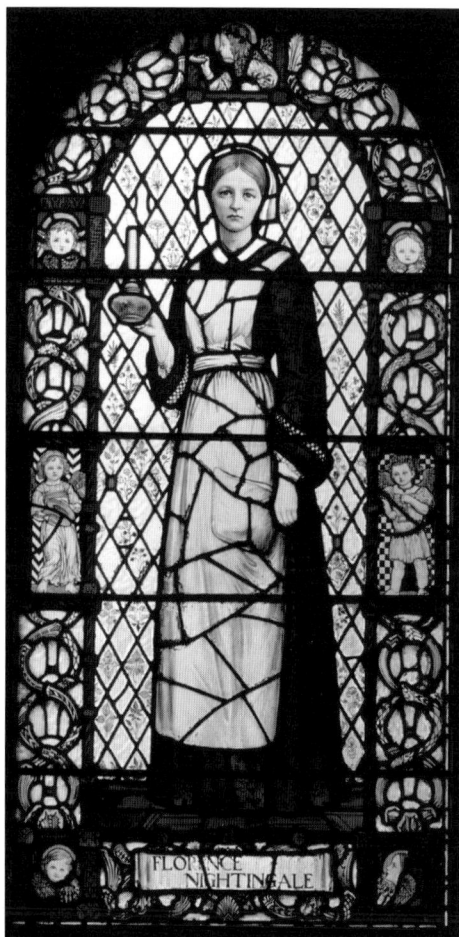

Left: Photo of Stained glass window- Florence Nightingale Glasgow Royal Infirmary chapel by Robert Anning Bell 1912. Presented by James D Hedderwick a manager of the Royal Infirmary 1912. (Courtesy of NHS Greater Glasgow and Clyde)

Below: A message from Florence Nightingale to Rebecca Strong. (Courtesy of NHS Greater Glasgow and Clyde)

A REPORT

OF THE ROYAL INFIRMARY OF GLASGOW, FROM ITS FIRST ESTABLISHMENT 8th. DECEMBER 1794, TILL 1st. JANUARY 1796,

FOR THE YEAR 1795.

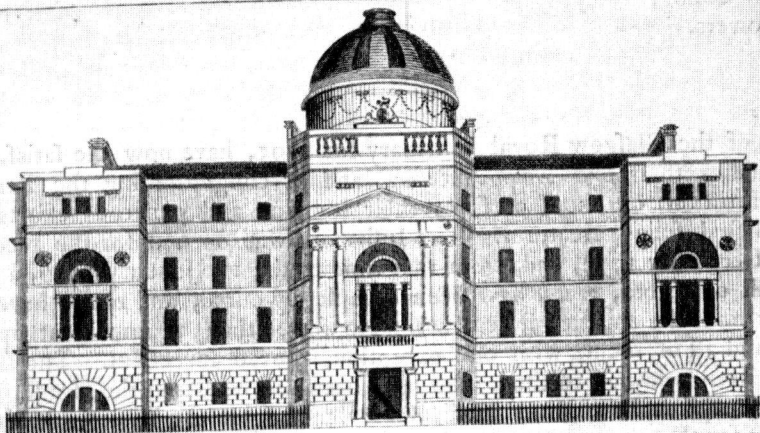

ROYAL Infirmary GLASGOW.

J. Haldane del.   et sculpsit.

LIST OF MANAGERS, 1795.

John Dunlop, Esq. Lord Provost,
William M'Dowall, Esq. M. P.
John Laurie, Esq. Dean of Guild,
William Auchinclofs, Esq. Deacon Convener,
Dr. Tho. Charles Hope, Professor of Medicine,
Dr. James Jeffray, Professor of Anatomy and
    Botany,
Dr. Cleghorn, in place of the President of the
    Faculty of Physicians and Surgeons,
Dr. Wright,
Dr. Taylor,
Messrs. David Dale,
    Robert Waddel,
    Archibald Grahame,

Messrs. John Stirling,
    Henry Riddel,
    John Buchanan,
    John Alston,
    Gilbert Hamilton,
    Walter Ewing M'Lae,
    William Wardlaw,
    William Couper,
    John Swanston,
    James Monteith,
    Archibald Smith,
    John Gordon.
    Professor Jardine,

A

Cover from 1st annual report, Glasgow Royal Infirmary 1794. (Courtesy of NHS Greater Glasgow and Clyde)

Regulations respecting the Admission of Patients, enacted by the General Court held on the first Monday of January, 1794.

1. That no Patient, excepting in cafes which do not admit of delay, fhall be admitted into the Infirmary, without the confent of a Committee to be appointed for that purpofe, of which Committee the attending Phyficians and Surgeons fhall be Members, but their number fhall not exceed one third of the Committee.

2. That Patients fhall be admitted by the recommendation of Contributors according to the following Rules.

3. That all Contributors of 10l. or more, or of 1l. 1s. or more, of annual Subfcription, may recommend one Patient annually.

4. That all Contributors of 20l. or more, or of 2l. 2s. or more, of annual Subfcription, may recommend Two Patients annually, but not have more than One Patient in the Infirmary at the fame time.

5. That all Contributors of 50l. or more, or of 3l. 3s. or more, of annual Subfcription, may recommend Four Patients annually, but not have more than One Patient in the Infirmary at the fame time.

6. That all Contributors of 100l. or more, or of 5l. 5s. or more, of annual Subfcription, may recommend Six Patients annually, but not have more than Two Patients in the Infirmary at the fame time.

7. That Incorporations or Societies, from which regular and perpetual recommendations may be expected, who have contributed 50l. or more, or 3l. 3s. of annual Subfcription, may recommend Two Patients annually, but not have more than one Patient in the Infirmary at the fame time.

8. That Incorporations, or Societies, who have contributed 100l. or more, or 5l. 5s. or more, of annual Subfcription, may recommend Four Patients annually, but not have more than Two Patients at the fame time in the Infirmary.

9. That Societies and Perfons who are both Contributors and annual Subfcribers, fhall be entitled to recommend both as Contributors and annual Subfcribers, according to the above Rules.

10. That Contributors fhall not be qualified to recommend till they fhall have paid their Contribution; nor annual Subfcribers, till they have paid their annual Subfcription one year.

11. That in all cafes of Competition in the recommendation of Contributors, or annual Subfcribers, a preference fhall be given to the priority of recommendation.

12. That fecurity fhall be given for defraying the expences of Burial, in cafe of death, which expence fhall be fixed at a moderate rate; and alfo, that the Patients be removed from the Infirmary when it is not proper they fhould continue longer there.

13. That the Servants of all Contributors, or Subfcribers, fhall be admitted into the Ward to be appropriated for fick or difeafed Servants, in preference to the Servants of Non-Subfcribers, and that the expences incurred during their continuance in the Infirmary fhall be fixed at a moderate rate.

14. That a book fhall be kept in which fhall be enrolled the names of the Patients, and the Subfcribers by whom they are recommended, the dates of their admiffion, and other particulars which the obfervation of the above Rules may require.

Niven, Napier, & Khull, Printers.

Regulation on admission of patients to Glasgow Royal Infirmary, 1794. (Courtesy of NHS Greater Glasgow and Clyde)

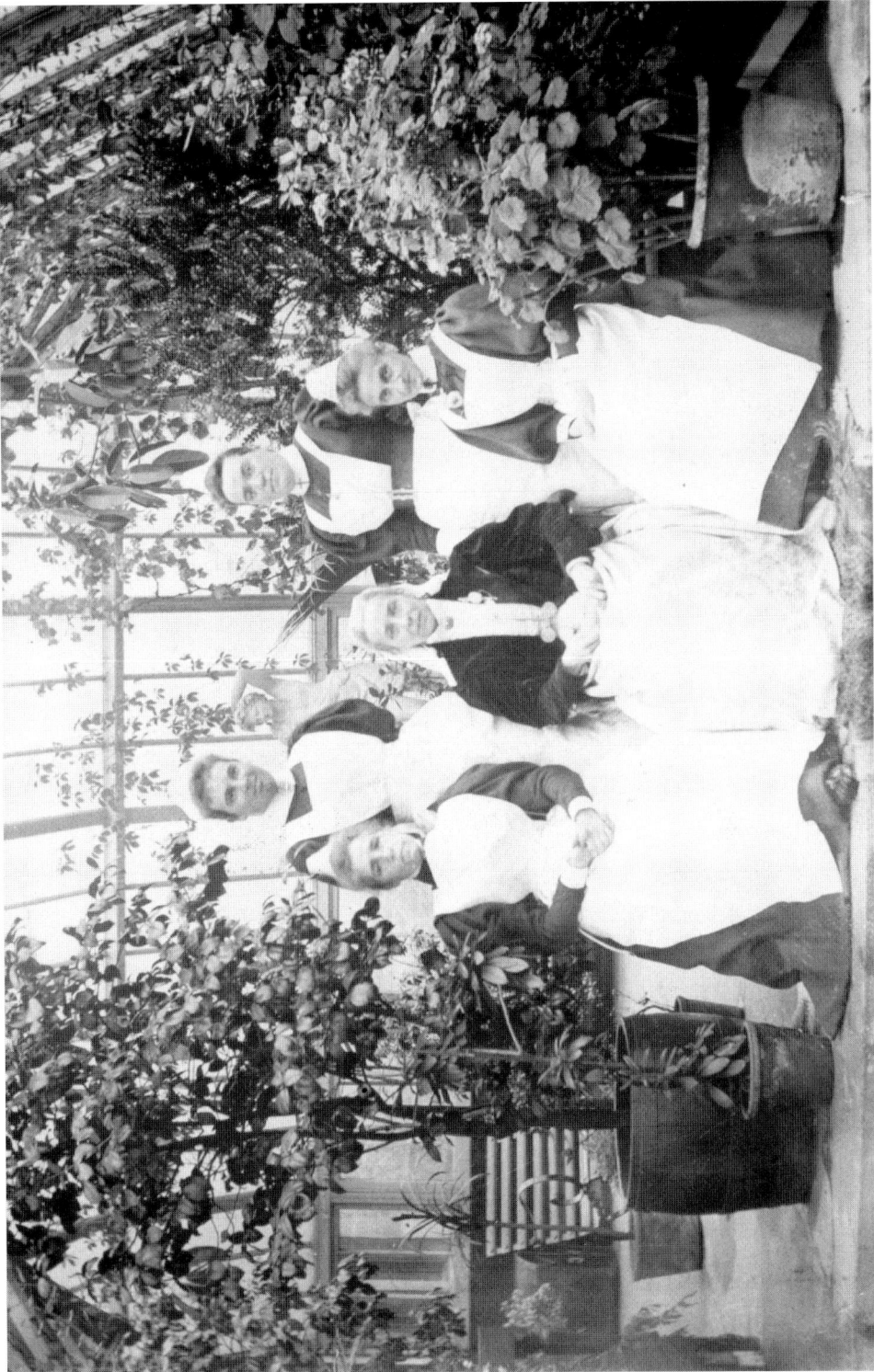

Rebecca Strong with Glasgow Royal Infirmary staff in conservatory, 1894. (Courtesy of NHS Greater Glasgow and Clyde)

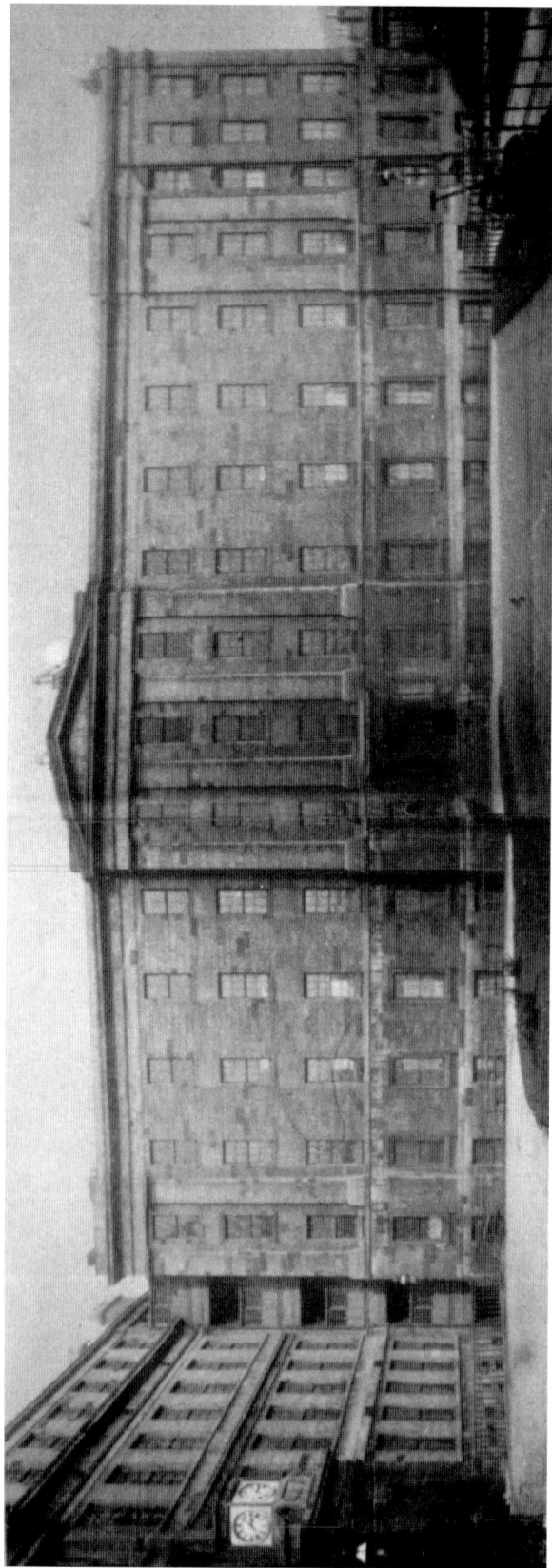

Glasgow Royal Infirmary, Old quadrangle showing Lister wards, 1890. (Courtesy of NHS Greater Glasgow and Clyde)

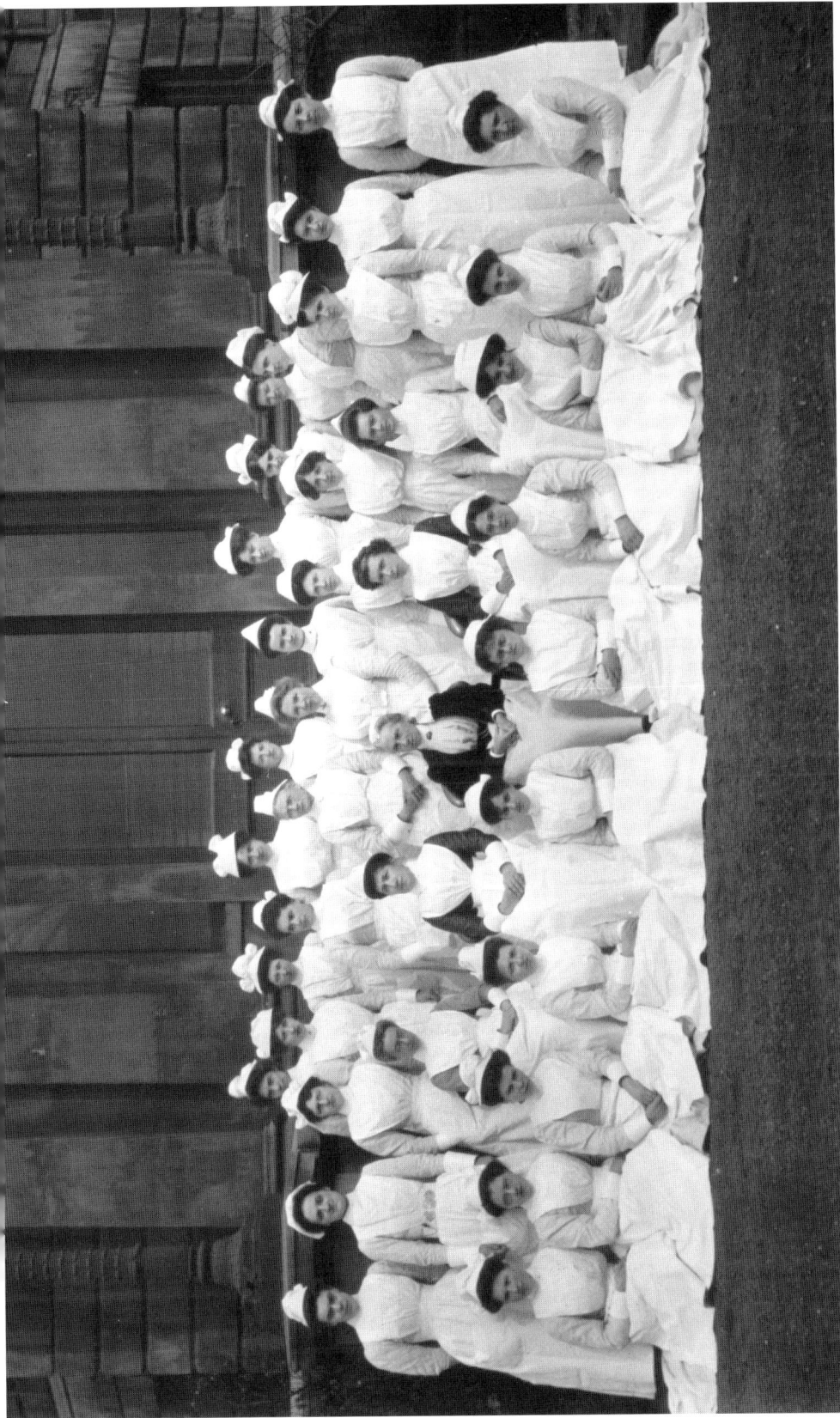

Rebecca Strong with group of nurses, Glasgow Royal Infirmary. (Courtesy of NHS Greater Glasgow and Clyde)

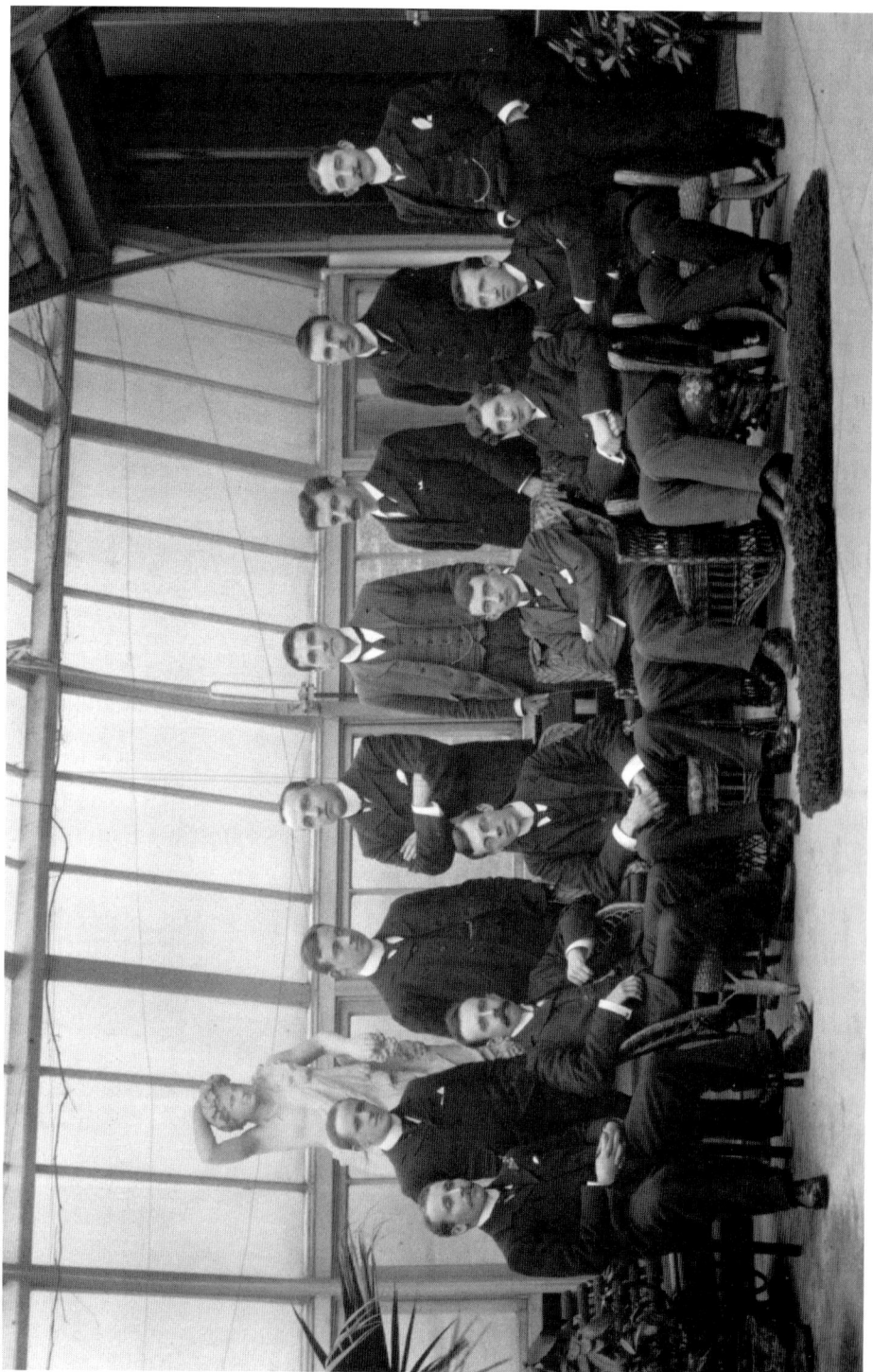

Glasgow Royal Infirmary Residents 1901 - Back row l to r Campbell Douglas, A. Gordon, F.H. Rainbird, H. Oswald-Smith, John W Leitch, Norman Sano, Hugh Campbell Ferguson. Front row l to r: C.M. Crawford, A.H. Watson, E.H. Roberts, Leonard Finlay, Thos B. Adam. (Courtesy of NHS Greater Glasgow and Clyde)

6.—**Drainage.** — Traps ; drains ; soil-pipe ; waste-pipe ; general principles of house drainage.

7.—**Water.**—Composition of pure water. Properties. Quantity required for different purposes. Common impurities and their effect on health. Hard and soft water. Diseases carried by water. Purification of water. Baths, varieties of—medicated baths, local baths, sponging. Bath-rooms; fittings; disposal of slops, excreta, &c.

8.—**Personal Hygiene.**—Regularity of habits. Exercise, outdoor and indoor. Mental recreation. Companionship; conversation; sleep; rest; holidays. Hereditary influence. Care of skin, teeth, nails, bowels.

9.—**Clothing.**—Materials employed and their properties. Functions of clothing. " Warmth " in clothing. Materials best adapted for under-clothing. Nurse's dress. Bedding and bed-clothing. Errors in dress.

10.—**Food** in relation to health.—Food in health and disease. Principles of invalid dietaries. Essentials of a healthy diet. Impurities in food; dangers to health from. Diseases carried by food.

11.—**Diseases.**—Definition of " epidemic," " endemic," " pandemic," " sporadic." Infection; contagion; inoculation. Bacteria in relation to disease. Incubation. Infective period. Segregation. Quarantine. Disinfection. The law in relation to infectious diseases.

12.—**Hospitals.**—Requirements according to cases to be treated. Reception of sick. Arrangement of wards. Special points as to lighting, heating, ventilation, decoration, &c.

Fee 2 guineas. Time 6 weeks. Non-resident.
Introduced 1893.

Text-books : " Hygiene for Students and Nurses," by Professor Glaister, M.D.; " Elements of Health," by Louis C. Parkes, M.D.

It is too much for any one to be occupied in ward work while studying these three subjects . Of course they require bringing up to date

Rebecca Strong

Syllabus for Glasgow Royal Infirmary nurse training with handwritten note from Rebecca Strong. (Courtesy of Royal College of Nursing Archives)

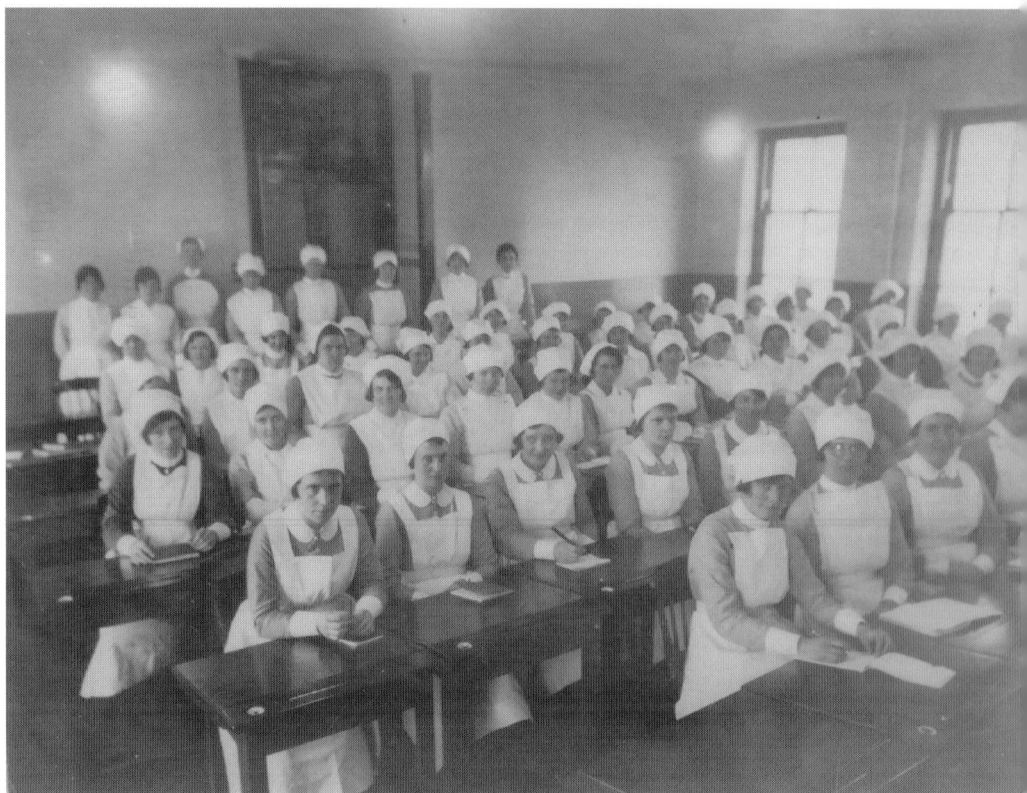

Nurses at lecture, Glasgow Royal Infirmary. (Courtesy Friends of Glasgow Royal Infirmary Museum)

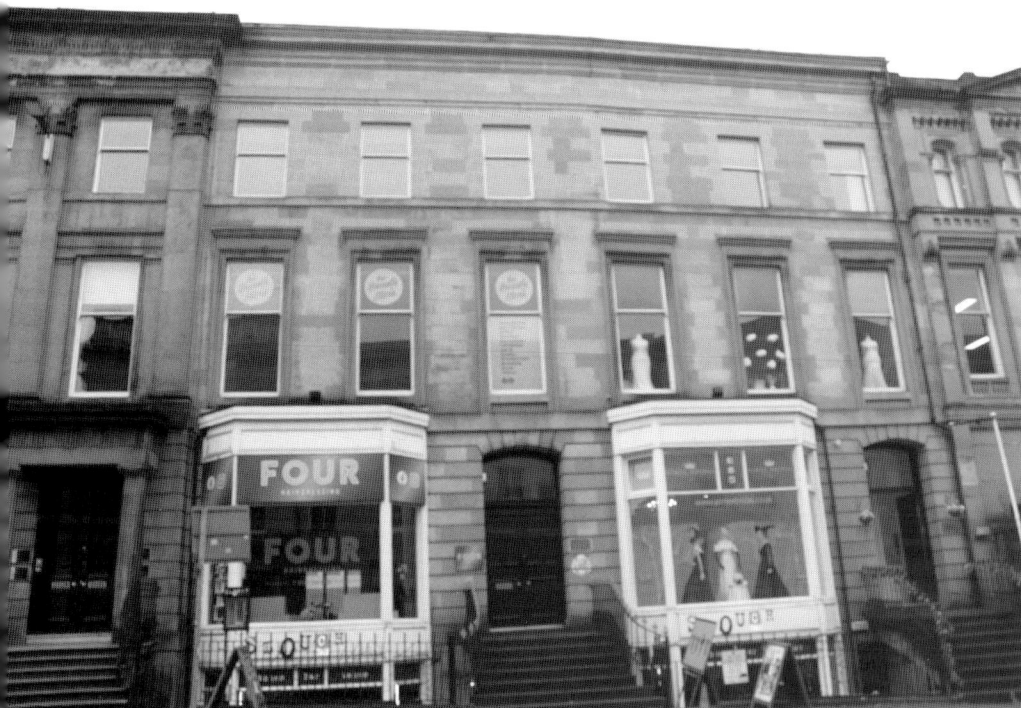

Above: Current view of 205 Bath Street, former premises of the Scottish Nurses' Club. (Judith Vallely)

Right: Sir William Macewen portrait, approx 1892. (Courtesy of NHS Greater Glasgow and Clyde)

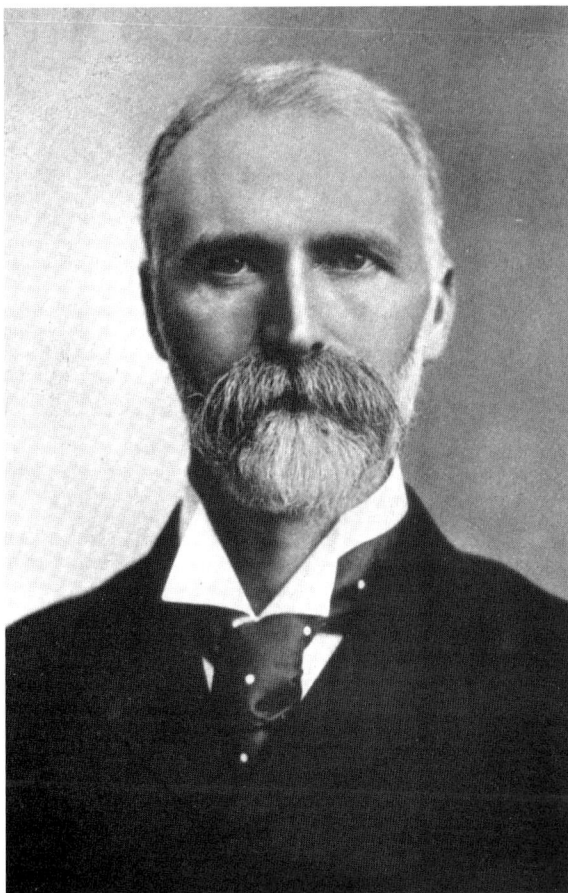

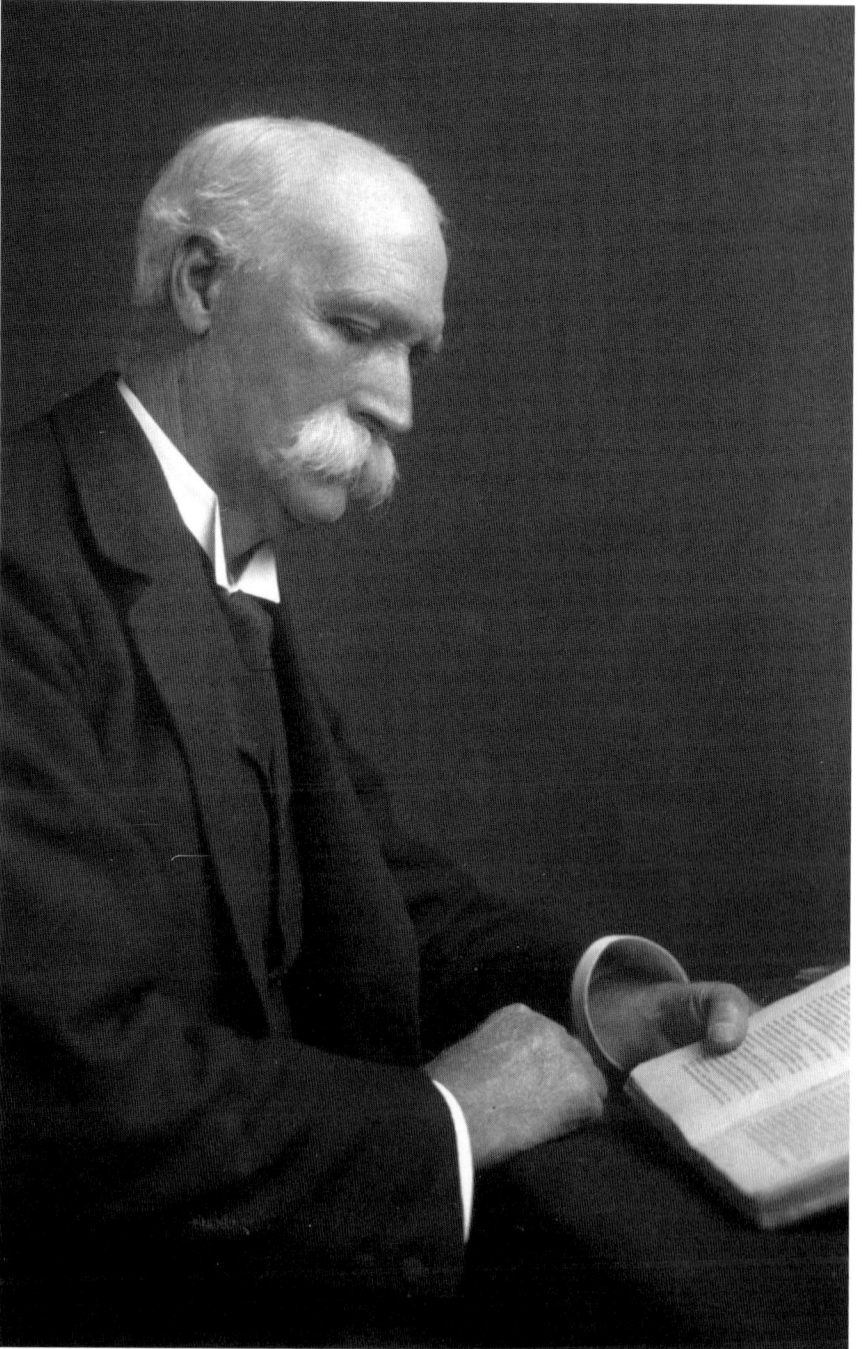

Sir William Macewen, portrait 1900. (Courtesy of NHS Greater Glasgow and Clyde)

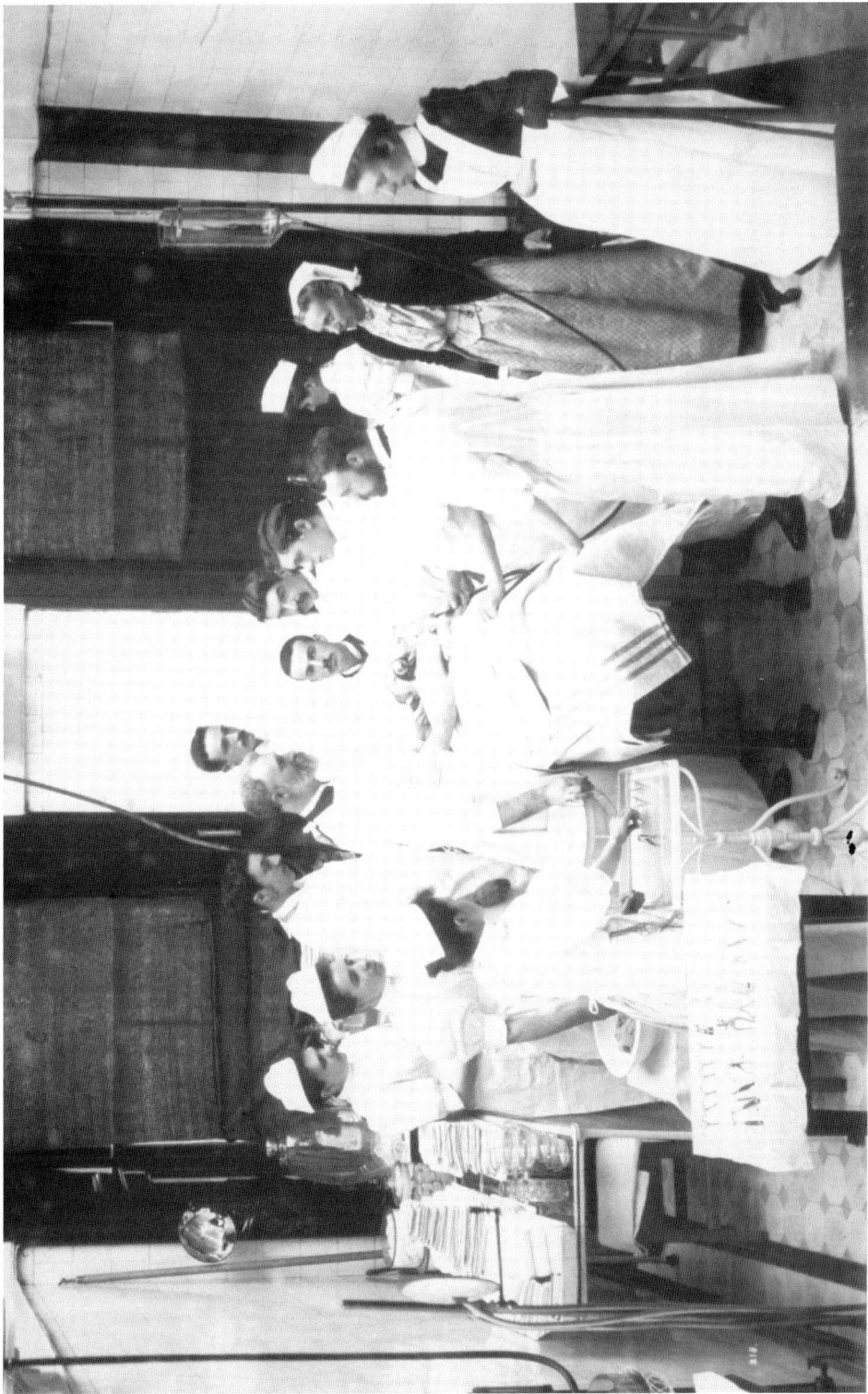

Rebecca Strong with William Macewen in operating theatre, Glasgow Royal Infirmary. (Courtesy of NHS Greater Glasgow and Clyde)

MARLBOROUGH HOUSE
S.W.1.

To Mrs Strong.
with best wishes
for your hundredth
birthday, from

Mary R

Aug 1943—

Left: Telegram from Queen Mary to Rebecca Strong, 1943. (Courtesy of NHS Greater Glasgow and Clyde)

Below: Telegram from King George V to Rebecca Strong, 1943. (Courtesy of NHS Greater Glasgow and Clyde)

Charges to pay			POST ☷ OFFICE		No. 139
s. d.					OFFICE STAMP
RECEIVED			TELEGRAM		
		Prefix. Time handed in. Office of Origin and Service Instructions. Words.			
From	m	9·0	Buckingham Palace 64	To	m
			OHMS.		

Mrs Rebecca Strong O.B.E.
Healthfield Vicars Cross Chester.
The Queen & I have heard with deep
interest of the lasting services which
you have rendered to the sick &
inspired by your great work in Nursing
On this your hundredth birthday from
which you look back over so many years

For free repetition of doubtful words telephone "TELEGRAMS ENQUIRY" or call, with this form B or C
at office of delivery. Other enquiries should be accompanied by this form and if possible, the envelope

Of tireless pioneering, we send
you our congratulations & best
wishes.
George R.I.

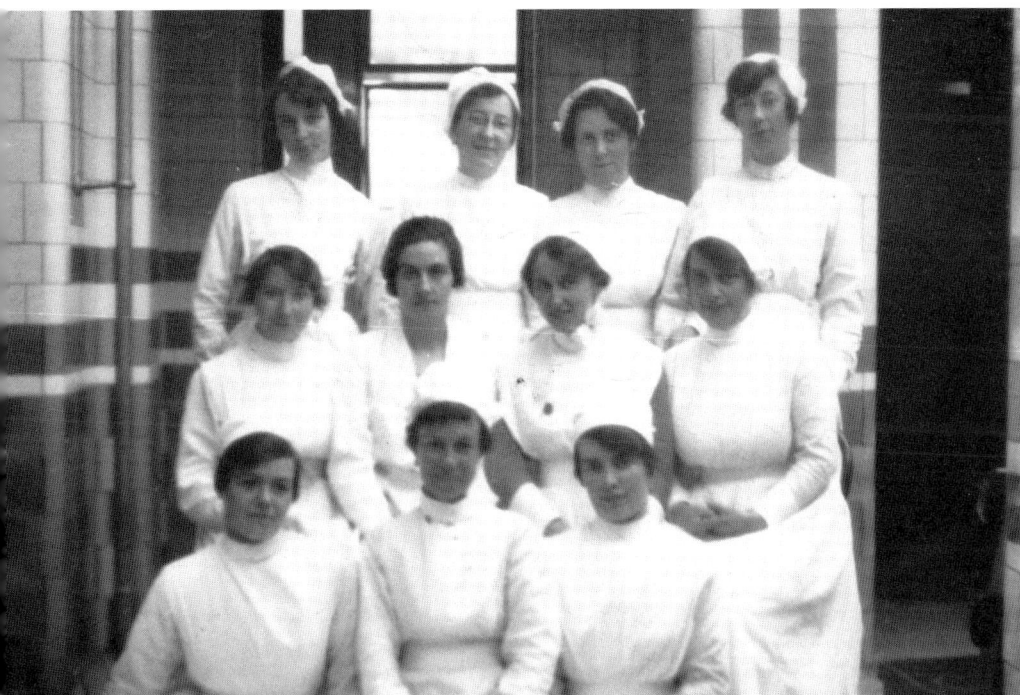

Glasgow Royal Infirmary nurses. (Courtesy of NHS Greater Glasgow and Clyde)

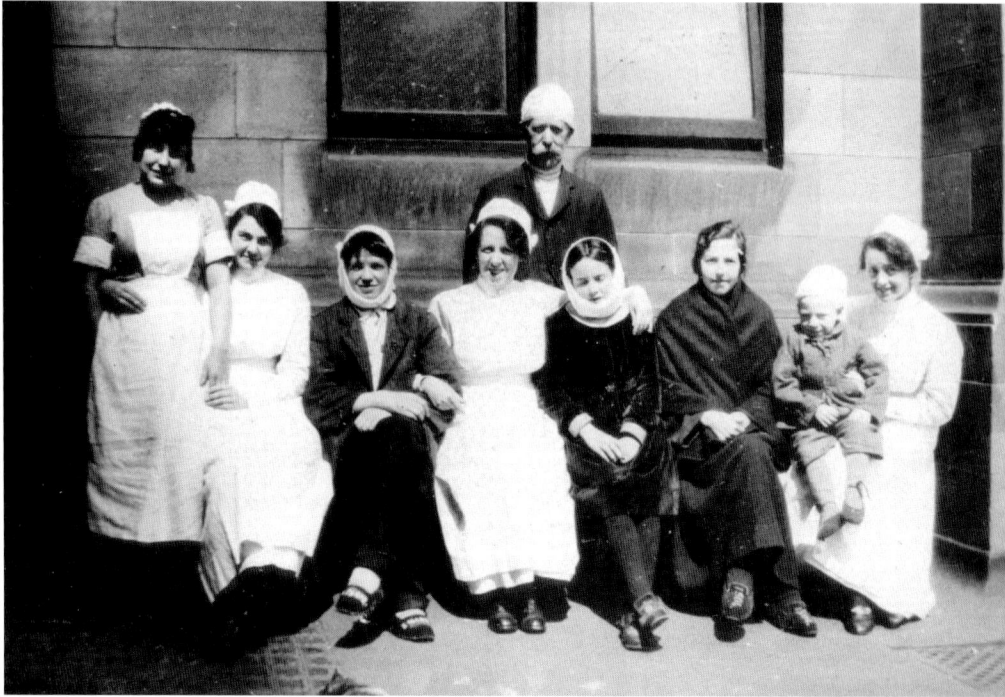

Glasgow Royal Infirmary nurses. (Courtesy of NHS Greater Glasgow and Clyde)

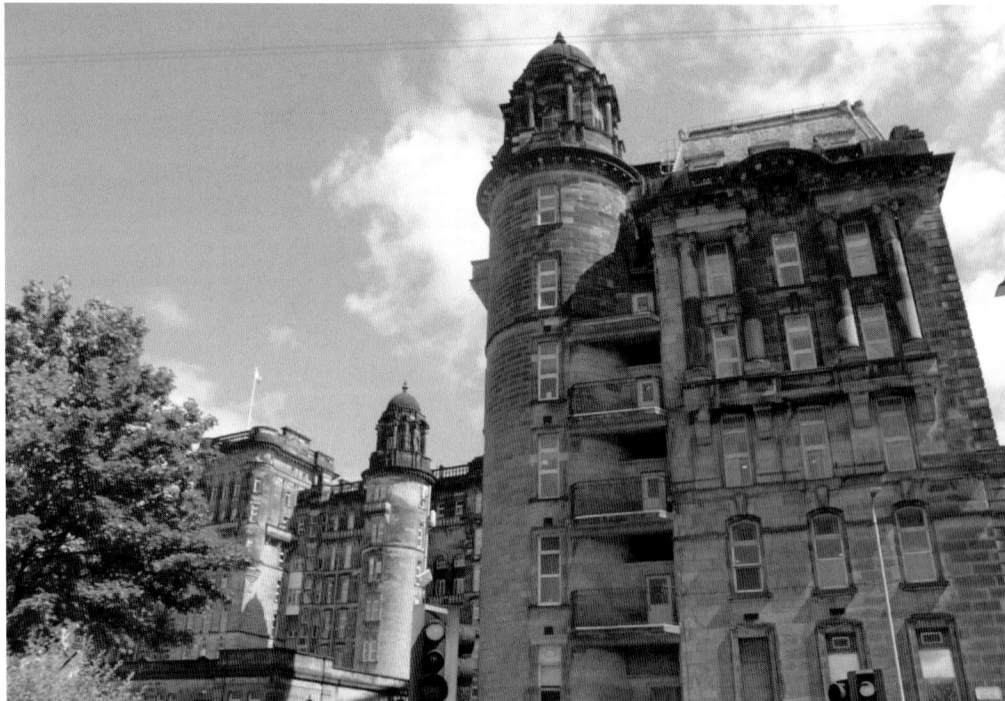

Current view of Glasgow Royal Infirmary. (Judith Vallely)

in favour of it being introduced. Strong was appointed as a member of the RBNA bill committee in the same year and her focus was on the nursing profession becoming self-governing, based on the idea of the proposed nursing council body being made up of a majority of independent nurses. She held a meeting of Scottish matrons to discuss the issue at Glasgow Royal Infirmary in November of that year.[3]

In 1909, two years after she had retired from Glasgow Royal Infirmary, Strong was elected to the General Council of the RBNA and appointed a member of the executive committee. In 1910, she was also made vice president of the National Council of Trained Nurses.[4]

Support for state registration for nurses was growing, but there were divisions over the best way to proceed. The Association for the Promotion of the Registration of Nurses in Scotland was formed in March 1909, but some supporters were in favour of Scotland forging its own way on a register, after a proposed English Registration Bill excluded Scotland. This was opposed by both Strong and Macewen and provoked strong reactions, as this letter in *The British Journal of Nursing* shows:

For some time it has been plain that two British Bills, differing only in minor points, are a hindrance to the passing into law of State Registration of Nurses by the Single Portal System. Many Scottish nurses signed for the Scottish Bill, unaware that it is a Bill out of which the vital principles of State Registration have been extracted. The Scottish Bill promotors simply sprang a Bill upon them, and they were whirled into it before they knew what they were doing. That a large number have extricated themselves from the net which was drawn in around them is well known, and now, when Sir William Macewen has taken the field, and it representing the party who are determined to fight for the Single Portal System for the United Kingdom of Great Britain and Ireland, the Society for State Registration and the Royal British Nurses' Association need have no fear that strong support will fail them from Scotland provided they ask Scottish nurses to support one British Bill. The Scottish Bill, as we know well – thanks to the outspoken manliness of Dr Wallace Anderson, an old and well-known friend of nurses – developed out of an anti-registration movement by a few medical men in Glasgow, and has at present the warm support of a publication edited by a lay male individual. In Scotland, we nurses who desire to see Registration upon a proper basis, class the promotors of the Scottish Bill with the Anti-Registration party.[5]

In the same edition of the journal, a report highlighted concerns about the impact of plans to exclude nurses trained in Scotland from the Nurses Registration Bill on those working south of the border:

If the Bill does not include Scotland, no nurse trained in a Scottish hospital can register until a Bill for Scotland is passed, so that their case would be a very difficult one. They could work as nurses, but would have no legal status, nor the right to the title of 'registered nurse'. In the case of private nurses, this would be specially unfortunate.[6]

However, it was not entirely a one-sided debate: there was support for the establishment of a separate registration system for nurses in Scotland:

Edinburgh Parish Council had before it on Monday a letter from Dr Mackintosh, Western Infirmary, Glasgow, as to the registration of nurses. It was stated that 2,718 nurses in Scotland are in favour of the establishment of a separate council for the registration of nurses in Scotland. Miss Brand, who had attended the meeting in Glasgow, said there was an almost unanimous feeling in favour of an independent separate system of registration for Scotland alone and apart from England. London was too far away, and the interests of Scottish hospitals and nurses might suffer. In the course of the discussion members expressed doubt as to whether nurses registered in Scotland would have an equal chance in England and Ireland.[7]

Macewen was part of a delegation from the Society of the State Registration of Nurses which travelled to see Prime Minister

Herbert Henry Asquith in May 1909, urging the government to enable a Bill to be introduced establishing a statutory council for the examination of trained nurses. In modern times, the system has so long been established it seems unlikely there would ever have be any arguments against it. But the delegation was only able to extract a promise from the prime minister that he would promise to give 'careful consideration' to their arguments due to pressure from opposed parties:

> Sir Victor Horsley spoke on behalf of the British Medical Association. The medical profession, he said, wished to see the nursing profession properly equipped. Mr Asquith, in reply, said so far as he could understand their desire was to promote the machinery for the examination of persons taking up the nursing profession, and to set up a register upon which those names could be subscribed. He pointed out that this would not in the least prevent other persons who had not satisfied the examiners from pursuing the profession of nursing. That was to say, a freelance would be just as able to carry on her profession as she was before. He had the views of persons who were entitled to the highest consideration, who were altogether opposed to the proposed legislation. These included many of the chairmen of London and provincial hospitals.[8]

Asquith also told the delegation he had received a list of names of 100 members of the medical profession in London, including some of the most eminent doctors – particularly the departments of obstetrics and surgery, and a list of 120 names 'in the provinces' – who were entirely opposed to the legislation proposed. There were 49 matrons of London hospitals, and 100 matrons of provincial hospitals, who were 'also entirely opposed'.

In July of that year, together with Strong, Macewen formed the Scottish Nurses' Association (SNA). The objectives of the SNA were set out as follows: to obtain state registration of nurses by a 'single portal system' for the United Kingdom, which would be extended, if possible, to the British Empire. It said the nurses were to be admitted to the register after three years' regulated training in recognised hospitals' schools, and having passed a state examination conducted under the auspices of a central board at suitable centres. Another stated aim was to raise and regulate the standards of education and training of nurses.

Macewen was appointed the first president, while Strong was named vice president and the creation of the association was welcomed in *The British Journal of Nursing*:

> There can be no question that organisation is urgently needed amongst Scottish nurses. At present they have no self-governing society, as English and Irish nurses have, through which to consider questions vital to their professional interests, or through which to take action. At no distant date trained nursing in the United Kingdom will be organised under the authority of a

Registration Council appointed by the State, and that registration scheme must affect Scottish nurses. It is imperative, therefore, they should find means of articulation, and this they cannot do as units ... Without a central professional body it is not possible to take effective action. This is to be the more regretted because Scottish nurses are of the best.

We warmly welcome the formation of the Scottish Nurses' Association. May it widen the scope of its objects, and add to its educational work the study of economic and humanitarian conditions.[9]

At the first annual meeting, in November 1909, Macewen gave an address and 'spoke of the need for the SNA to promote the dignity of nursing as a profession and to obtain a distinguishing title for its graduates. He drew attention to the unsatisfactory position of nurses in Britain compared to the colonies and on the continent, where state registration was already in practice.'[10]

Strong had become more involved with the SNA after her sister died and she had moved back to Scotland. She was appointed president of the organisation and with the outbreak of the First World War and a shortage of trained nurses, argued a standard qualification for the profession was needed more urgently than ever before.

In 1916, the College of Nursing was established – but Strong was initially critical of it as yet another voluntary system of registration, rather than the model of state registration with a statutory General Nursing Council, which she saw as the gold standard. In the autumn of that year, she outlined her views as she gave the opening address at a conference held by the National Union of Trained Nurses:

> She welcomed the impetus which the arrival of the College of Nursing had given the long-standing cause of uniformity in nurses' education. Nevertheless, she criticised the proposed rules of the College which would accept nurses for registration from recognised training schools and leave the majority of the smaller schools ostracised. Her contention was that a minimum standard of theoretical knowledge should be set by examination, so that training in hospitals, large or small, could be tested and a common diploma awarded, thus placing all hospitals on the same footing. Her preference was for the term 'graduate in nursing' rather than registered nurse.[11]

Addressing a meeting of the National Council of Trained Nurses in 1916, Strong said she wanted to see it made illegal for anyone to enter a hospital for practical training without having a specific course of training beforehand and to see nurses form a governing body for themselves:

> You know, or should know, your own needs. If you have clear thought you will have clear speech. Make up your minds what it is you want and stick to it.[12]

The divisions over the best way to introduce state registration continued. The idea of a joint bill, initially put forward by the College of Nursing and the Central Committee for State Registration of Nurses, broke down in 1916, to be replaced by a focus on separate bills. But the issue ground to a halt due to the ban on Private Members' Bills introduced during the war and no progress was made until this was lifted. In 1919, the two Bills were introduced in the House of Commons and the House of Lords:

> Both Bills had their supporters and their critics in the two Houses. The Association for the Promotion of Registration of Nurses in Scotland issued a memorandum, signed by 59 matrons and nurses, criticising the Central Committee's Bill as partisan and attacking the Scottish Nurses' Association as a local Glasgow society with no following in Edinburgh. The College of Nursing also criticised the Central Committee's Bill for the unjust representation it gave on the proposed general nursing council to the various nurses' societies. No agreement had been reached when Parliament rose in July, and when it resumed in the autumn, the Minister of Health introduced a government Bill for the registration of nurses.[13]

The bill was passed as the Nurses' Registration Act on 23 December 1919, and the first General Nursing Council (GNC) for England and Wales was established the following year, with similar bodies also set up in Scotland and Ireland. The government had argued different registers were needed as the administration of public health was distinct for these countries.

The GNC for England and Wales set out the requirements that to be admitted to the register, nurses had to be over 21, provide three references of good character and have at least one year's training and two years of practice prior to November 1919. A committee was also created which had the power to discipline nurses who were found to have breached standards.

The register opened in September 1921 with Ethel Gordon Fenwick becoming the first to sign as 'state registered nurse number one'. The achievement of the goal of registration was therefore fresh in her mind when Strong addressed a reunion of Glasgow Royal Infirmary nurses in December 1921, comprising 'a large and representative gathering drawn from every generation of nurses since 1879' when she had been appointed matron of the hospital. She spoke of the significance of the setting up of the register:

> I do not think that such a gathering as this should be without a mention of Mrs Bedford Fenwick's name. I do not think that anyone has given more – herself and her money for the advancement of the nursing profession – than Mrs Bedford Fenwick. She began the battle thirty years ago, in the face of opposition from many London Matrons, and you must not misunderstand me, even of

Miss Nightingale. Miss Nightingale said that in forty years' time probably Registration would be required, if our Hospitals kept up the level, and Nurses made the best use of their time, but fortunately we have got it in thirty years. If it had not been for Mrs Bedford Fenwick we would not have had Registration today.

Strong said while the Registration Bill had now been passed, the nurses had to remember they were only at the 'beginning of things' and not the end, as she urged them to continue fighting to improve the profession:

Do not lose your individuality. Form your ideals and stick to them, and let them be noble ones. Do not allow the idea to get into your work that when the bell rings, you automatically stop work. In the olden days we never thought about hours; we often were on duty night and day. The best, however, is not got out of nurses under these conditions – the patients suffer, your health suffers – therefore your hours must be regulated. Above all, do not let yourselves become machines; keep your souls as well as your bodies in health. Keep yourselves interested, as the more interested you are the better qualified you are for your work. Unless every faculty is cultivated you will not make good nurses. The mental needs of your patients must be considered as well as the physical. When man is ill – I mean man in the large term – his sensitiveness is highly increased, and if you are tired mentally or physically, your patient will at once know. My final word to you all is – Keep your Ideals.

Five years later, addressing a meeting of the Scottish Nurses' Association as president, she also spoke of the significance of registration:

> There has been much clamour for professional status, and it has been gained … When this great Gift came I hailed it with joy, as nursing had made such rapid strides of late, and there are so many important positions, unthought of a few years ago, which require higher education, and which by the help of bursaries, scholarships, etc., will be open to those who have the brain power to attain them.[14]

Today, nursing and midwifery in England, Scotland, Wales and Northern Ireland is regulated by one body, the Nursing and Midwifery Council (NMC). As well as maintaining the register, it promotes high education and professional standards and has a code which sets out expected standards and behaviour, with the powers to investigate allegations about the fitness to practise of individuals. The latest annual data from the NMC showed a record number of nurses, midwives and nursing associates were on the register in 2022–2023 – equivalent to 1.2 per cent of the estimated UK population.[15]

The SNA, which had been co-founded by Strong, was also key in setting up a popular club for nurses based in Glasgow.

In March 1917, premises for the Scottish Nurses' Club were secured initially at two rooms in 103 Bath Street in the city and Strong, who had been living in Perthshire, moved to Glasgow to supervise the refurbishment of the rooms. For a small subscription, nurses – including those in training – were able to access a room for reading and writing and 'conversation purposes', with discussions on nursing politics encouraged:

> The rooms proved very popular, over 400 nurses joined within a few months, and the idea of extending the accommodation to provide a proper nurses' club was considered. The Lord Provost of Glasgow, Sir Thomas Dunlop, offered his official help and an appeal was launched as the City's tribute to nurses for their war work. Over £10,000 was raised within six months and the trustees of the fund were able to purchase premises at 205 Bath Street, which became the home of the Scottish Nurses' Club for many years.[16]

The club at 205 Bath Street, which consisted of a drawing and a dining room, a library, twenty-one bedrooms and a kitchen and a stove, was officially opened on 14 December 1918:

> The Club, located in one of the most beautiful houses in Bath Street, is largely the outcome of the work for the nursing profession of Mrs Strong, late Matron of

the Royal Infirmary, Glasgow, and President of the
Scottish Nurses' Association, a pioneer worker for the
nursing profession who is still in the van of progress ...
Perhaps no body of workers need a professional Club,
or appreciate it more, than trained nurses, who, whether
they live in hospitals or are engaged in private nursing,
or in branches of social service, long for a home of their
own, for the best women are by instinct home-makers,
and one of the trials of a nurse's life is that so seldom has
the opportunity of exercising that instinct. The Club is
appointed with great taste and is most comfortably, and
indeed, luxuriously furnished. To spend their off-duty
time in harmonious surroundings is to many nurses a
greater rest that is often understood, for beautiful form
and perfectly blended colours are not only an enjoyment
but a real rest to nerves which are constantly at tension
during duty hours.[17]

During the opening ceremony, Strong gave the vote of thanks
and a short address to the nurses:[18]

This Club is a most noble gift, one which I hope will
mean the parting of the ways out of the old net of
narrowness of view and of spirit into the open ground
of fellowship and goodwill – not school against school.
Great as the gift is, it is only the foundation stone, the
superstructure lies with yourselves. The whole country
has been roused out of its listless, selfish, indifferent

attitude towards things in general. Take your share in this new spirit, listen to the best that is in you, and see that you leave a goodly heritage both of word and deed. If we begin on right lines developments will take place, evolution being one of the laws of life. Whatever we may do will only meet the demands of the moment, fresh demands will arise with fresh needs, whenever we think we have attained, we shall begin to deteriorate.

Strong said she hoped the nurses' club would be an educational centre as well as a place of recreation – saying that now women have the power of voting, one evening in week should be given to the study of politics and general subject which 'affect the general welfare of mankind'. She went on:

The nurses of the Public Health Department of Glasgow, who have by means of a concert and otherwise raised £120, desire the sum to be spent upon library furnishings and books, further donations will be acceptable as we want a library of good professional as well as general literature. I also hope that our staunch friends of the medical profession will give post graduate lectures so that nurses who have left hospital may be kept in touch with the modern methods of treatment. Those of you who are commencing your career are doing so under exceptionally favourable circumstances when the feeling of brotherhood is abroad in a greater measure than ever before, and amongst testimonies of recognition of service this beautiful Club will testify to the generosity of the citizens of Glasgow in giving practical acknowledgement of the services rendered by Scottish Nurses in the hour of our country's need. We must not forget the return of our nurses from the battle fronts which will shortly occur; many of them, weary in body and mind, worn out with witnessing such sights as I hope the world may never again see. I sincerely trust that some means may be devised of giving them a helping hand during the period of waiting before they are fit for, or can obtain, fresh employment.

The premises were given a glowing review in *The British Journal of Nursing*, which noted that the club is 'centrally situated and very accessible, thanks to the excellence of the tramway service of Glasgow':

The sitting room gives at once an impression of spaciousness and restfulness for it is most harmoniously and artistically decorated and furnished, the colour scheme being one of soft fawn, blending into brown relieved by a touch of pink. The members greatly appreciate this charming room, and the opportunity it offers them of rest as well as of access to the daily papers, thus keeping them in touch with the outside world. But an equal boon to nurses is that they can here receive their friends and offer them hospitality for the sitting room opens into a lofty, well-lit restaurant in the same tone of colouring. Here, at very moderate cost, most tempting meals are to be obtained.[19]

Strong was associated with the club for many years, both as a trustee and as a welcome speaker.[20] The Scottish Nurses' Club was still at the Bath Street premises in the 1940s, with archive pictures held by Historic England showing nurses playing a game of bridge in one of the rooms. In 1943, a message of congratulations was read at the club's annual meeting from Queen Mary at a meeting which also noted, with a total of 1,097 weekly residents, the previous year had been the busiest in the club's history:

> Expressing her deep concern in the welfare of the nursing service and interest in every step which is taken to improve salaries and conditions, Queen Mary voiced the hope that, with the inducement of improved salaries and conditions, more women will enter the nursing profession, and that nurses who have retired or married will take up nursing again. She sincerely hoped that with such improvements there would be a large increase in the number of candidates for the nursing profession.

Today the building which housed the Scottish Nurses' Club is still in existence – at the time of writing, a bridal shop was located in the premises.

Chapter Eight

Dear William Macewen …

Acclaimed Scottish surgeon Sir William Macewen, born in the Isle of Bute, was a supporter of Strong's ideas and a friend to her, as highlighted in previous chapters. He became renowned for performing the world's first successful operation to remove a brain tumour – saving the life of a teenage girl – which took place at Glasgow Royal Infirmary in 1879.[1]

During his student days, he trained under Joseph Lister, whose pioneering use of antiseptics formed the basis of modern infection control and Macewen was one of the first surgeons to adopt his methods, as well as developing the technique further. Dr Kate Stevens, co-founder of the charity Friends of Glasgow Royal Infirmary, points to this as being a key aspect of his backing for Strong – he needed to have the best nursing staff around him to ensure his antisepsis techniques were applied:

> It didn't matter how clean he was – if he was using gloves and carbolic acid – if the nurses were dirty and drunk, the surgery wasn't really going to be a success.[2]

Macewen had been appointed as full surgeon at Glasgow Royal Infirmary in 1877, at the age of 29. He was in charge of three wards and known for working continuously and demanding high standards of his nurses, who were relied upon to make detailed observations of his patients to alert him to the slightest change in their condition.

But the relationship was not without its ups and downs, with Strong often seeking to protect her nurses amid Macewen's high demands, as demonstrated in correspondence between the pair. A series of letters preserved by descendants of Macewen are held in the archives of the Royal College of Physicians and Surgeons of Glasgow. The correspondence was written over the course of eighteen months, and is mainly from Strong to Macewen – but does shed some fascinating light on the relationship between the two.

An analysis of the letters, written by Tom Gibson, notes that when the first of the letters was written Strong was 38 years old and Macewen was four years her junior, with the surgeon in charge of three wards at Glasgow Royal Infirmary – 21, 22 and 29:

> Both needed the other: Macewen performing new operations under strict asepsis needed intelligent, trainable nurses to tend his patients. Mrs Strong needed Macewen, a surgeon already of great international renown, to help forward her plans.[3]

In the first letter, dated 9 January 1882, Strong referred to concerns over the health of the nurses in ward 22 – indicating that they have been previously 'overtaxed':

I have no probationer ready until March 1st. If this new one is not actually in the way during your visit I shall feel obliged by your allowing her to remain in the ward merely to assist the nurses. To keep the children thoroughly clean & do all the work that is required of them in 22 is really too much for the nurses continuously. The health of the 3 considerably improved after the lessening of the work and it seems a pity to overtax them again.

A month later, she wrote to Macewen urging him to be more aware of the conditions in which his night nurses were having to work – warning they appeared to be tired after working twelve-hour shifts in which they had to be constantly alert:

When speaking to you last evening I quite forgot to put in a word for your night nurses. They have made no complaint, but I notice that they appeared a good deal fatigued. If at any time I ask, if they are going out regularly, I invariably receive some such answers as this – 'Well you see it is difficult, Dr Macewen's visit is generally a long one, & he does not like us to leave & if we ask to do so, we are afraid he will think we have no interest in our work.' They dine at 12.30 & then to bed. The hours for sleep are short enough, they are called at 9. Night duty is not what it used to be. There is no taking of sleep during the night. All easy chairs are strictly forbidden and they have to be on the alert the whole night. 12 consecutive hours of this (from 10 till 10) is very fatiguing. I speak from experience. It is a hard & fast rule that no nurse goes out on receiving day, excepting by special permission. If you can see your way to relieve them a little more on the other four days I think it will benefit them very much.

The letters reveal how pressure continued to build during this year – which was during Strong's first rather difficult tenure as matron at Glasgow Royal Infirmary. In April, she wrote to Macewen over fears that they were approaching a 'misunderstanding' following a clash with one of his assistants over who should be giving the orders to nurses.[4]

She described an incident in which she told a Nurse McDonald to sit beside a patient in the side room of ward 22 – but when another member of staff went to fetch her. the nurse refused, saying she took her orders from resident medic Dr David Potts. In a letter to Macewen. Strong said that when she quizzed her, the nurse stated Potts told her to disobey the matron – which Strong noted was the second occurrence of its kind:

The previous one was with Nurse Dewing. I saw you on Sunday afternoon, telling you, Nurse Dewing felt the work too much for her and that I would send Nurse Fraser the following morning to you. Dr Potts was engaged in the ward at the time & it was not convenient for me to speak to him. In the evening Nurse Dewing came to me, saying, Dr Potts told her she was not to go. I told her to change & I would make the matter right, whereupon I sent an explanatory note to Dr Potts. I leave you to judge whether it is seemly, even in the event of a blunder, to have my instructions disputed. To govern 90 women under the most favourable circumstances is not an easy task. I think it is almost a mistake on your part to ask me to make any arrangements for the nursing of your patients beyond supplying you with 10 nurses ... I think it would be much better if you would arrange the work with your Assistant & leave him to give the orders. I should not like to subject myself a third time to having my orders contradicted & if I have the giving of them, there is again the possibility of my doing so without the knowledge of your Assistant.

There is also an added PS to the letter, which said: 'Whether it is good for the morale of the house to leave arrangements in the hands of the Assistants is a matter of opinion.'

Tensions clearly continued to build, as illustrated by a letter Strong wrote on 19 May 1882 which described her growing fury and indicated that she was thinking about leaving her post:

I am desperately angry today at being asked to supply another probationer for ward 22, especially after having already supplied an extra one for 29. I do not see how a nurse in the place is to get a holiday if none of them are able to do a bit of extra work. It certainly reflects badly on the management of 22 if the nurse cannot manage for a short time with three nurses the same as the other wards. I heartily repent putting the second probationer into 22 as I certainly meant her to be the means of relieving the pressure of work in your three wards ... 22 has so monopolised the services of the two probationers that they feel themselves ill-used immediately they have only one. I told them today I was thoroughly disgusted, especially after their getting up a memorial for my remaining – that words costs nothing, but the moment a bit of extra service was required from them they were ill-used. If they would only act like sensible women and go to their beds in proper time instead of hanging about all hours of the night & day (requiring to be hunted up like children) they would be capable of a good deal more work. I have come to the conclusion that the more you do for people, the more you may & no thanks for it ... What with watching cases, and sick nurses we happen to be particularly hampered, so much so that I shall have to give my services tonight.

She ended with a scathing remark: 'I heartily pity the poor wretch that comes after me and hail my own exit with delight.'

In August of the same year, she raised concerned over the relationship which had emerged between one of the nurses and Potts. She also revealed that she had submitted her resignation – with managers setting up a special committee to investigate her complaints over her authority being undermined:

Nurse Walker has this morning told me of her engagement to Dr Potts & suppose this to be the 'other cause' you alluded to. All appears to be perfectly honourable & therefore nothing can be said about it, only I think he should have spoken out long before & one of them left the house. I cannot understand a man exposing the woman he wishes to marry to any kind of slander. I had thorough faith in the characters of both or the rumours that reached me would not have passed unheeded. My resignation went in on Thursday. A Special Committee meet tomorrow to consider the matter and I have been asked to put in writing any explanations I wish to make. The substance of what I have said is that the assistant Drs are too young and inexperienced to have the full control of the nursing arrangements in their respective wards & to secure the good working of the house, the visiting 'Medical Staff' should communicate directly with myself. Do not think I slight your comment or undervalue your advice: under the circumstances I think it better for you not to be in any way involved & wish to be able to say that I have asked quite unadvisedly.[5]

The subcommittee that was set up found there were differing views on the management of staff between Strong and the hospital's superintendent, who was her direct superior. He considered the matron was too inflexible when it came to young resident medical staff, while she believed he was not strict enough, leading to subordination. The threat of Strong's departure was, in the end, averted by the findings of the investigation:

> The committee agreed with Mrs Strong's view, and decided that the Superintendent had not adequately supported her position and authority and recommended that the distribution of the nurses and probationers should be in the hands exclusively of the Matron, with power of review only with the Superintendent. Since this was the arrangement which Mrs Strong had requested, she agreed to withdraw her resignation.[6]

But the crisis was only temporarily solved. In November of that year, Strong handed in her notice again – then subsequently withdrew it following a fortnight's rest. Four letters, all written within a fortnight, show her escalating concerns, with references to difficulties around Miss Purchase and Miss Corran who were the Superintendents of Nursing under Strong:

> In Dr Dunn's zeal to serve you, he forgot there was a certain amount of courtesy required & that whatever his personal dislike to Miss Purchase may be, it does not do to allow it to interfere with work. When Miss

Purchase asked Nurse Dewing to remain until one and Dr Dunn openly contradicted her and said ND was not to stay, Miss P went to Miss Corran and asked advice. Miss C advised her to stand her ground & keep Nurse D until one & then either find someone else or stay herself, Miss P preferred staying, knowing we were shorthanded. That extra nurse in your wards has cost me more than I ever calculated for, although I calculated a good deal. From the height of the wards & the messages to be done, I still think it necessary to have her there. There has been far less knocking up amongst your nurses since you had an extra hand & that speaks for itself. I think I may safely undertake to meet all emergencies as I have done in the past & sincerely hope I shall never require to meet you officially again.

In a letter dated 15 November 1882, Strong wrote to Macewen that she was thankful to have spoken to him the previous night and 'got rid of that dreadful feeling of officialism' – and said that she hoped that she would never have to meet with him in an 'official capacity' again. Two days later, she penned another note to Macewen which said she was sorry if 'any arrangement has been made of which you do not approve'. With only Strong's letters surviving, it is of course not clear what this relates to – but she does urge him to consult with other staff members and 'make any arrangements you wish'.

The letter added: 'I am fairly knocked up with worries – not work – and go off today for a fortnight. I was trying hard to hold out until April when I go altogether but could not manage it.'[7]

Strong continued the correspondence when she was aboard the Belfast boat and the longest letter, which is part of the preserved series, appears to be a pouring out of all that is troubling her. Reading the letter, it is possible to imagine her sitting on the boat listening to the sounds of the sea and reflecting on her job at Glasgow Royal Infirmary and wondering whether it was possible to continue:

In the quietness of the night I wonder what the mystery of the past week has been. Everything in your wards seems to have gone wrong. I cannot think it is simply in consequence of Nurse Wendy having but 6 hours rest in one 24 hours – or Nurse Dewing being asked to remain on duty until 1 a.m. I have no doubt in my present state of health I may be unduly sensitive & apt to magnify evils. I felt you were at enmity with me and simply could not endure it after your true friendship towards me & suddenly made my mind up to go away for a fortnight, hoping things will right themselves a little in that time. I know it is cowardly. I had better speak out what I think; it seems to me as if your mind were being poisoned by some one and if your own judgement after a three & half years knowledge of me cannot stand its ground, then I must experience all the bitterness of a misplaced confidence. I have quite made up my mind that April is to see the last of me in the

GRI. I did not think it possible to have laboured so much as I have done & been so much misunderstood. What I do revel in, is the thankful hearts of those good old nurses & the parting with them will be a trial.

There is another section of the letter written in pencil, in which she says she had to retire with a 'perturbed stomach'. She appeared to have then reflected on what she had written, saying it may be a 'distorted view' – but added she will allow it to remain:

It is now 6 a.m. and we are waiting to get into harbour. I do not think you can have peace in your wards unless some arrangement can be made whereby one and only one receives your instructions for arrangements. I do think that one should be the Matron's assistant & she should be directly responsible to you for the carrying of them out. Your assistant is always with you & you could tell him of any arrangements you are to make. I speak purely for the good of your wards & not through any personal feeling.

My decision is irrevocable and it will not affect me either way. At present it is most confusing. Sometimes you tell arrangements to Miss Corran, sometimes myself, sometimes Dr Dunn & sometimes Mary. If the Matron's assistant gives instructions to the nurses for the different wards in which they are to be placed it establishes her position with them, bringing her into closer contact & causing them to look up to her. This is a widely different thing from receiving instructions for the treatment of patients. It would be madness to think of her receiving those.

The last section of this letter was written on notepaper with the embossed crest of the Belfast Hospital for Sick Children with the observation it was 8.30 a.m. and Strong was back on 'terra firma'. She appears to have been appealing to Macewen to reassure her over a dispute which arose over arrangements for the nurses on the wards:

Nurse Wendy going to 29 ward was suggested by me & sanctioned by you to Miss Corran. I was anxious for her to be as useful to you in the Children's Hospital & knew she could gain much more information in 29 than any other ward. The whole of her surgical work has been amongst children. We have been so accustomed to a pleasant look & word from you we cannot understand anything else, & yet of course as in all lives there must be numberless anxieties of which we can know nothing. I would fain lighten them if I could, instead of adding to them. I should be glad to have a line from you to say if I have done anything to offend you. Our number of nurses will be made up on Monday & you can get a little more help if the need still remains. I do think you were a little hard on me. I am accustomed to it with the rest of the house but not with you. It would be quite easy for me to take the first woman who offers herself when a vacancy occurs. If I can get a better by waiting for a few days I prefer doing so. I am sorry to miss the opportunity of meeting yourself and Mr Sellars. I am glad he had the good sense not to lose the opportunity. The hearing of the discussion would have been useful as well as pleasant. I shall be moving about but a note addressed to c/o Mrs Chambers, Mill Road Hospital, Liverpool, will find me.

Whatever Macewen wrote back, it seems to have provided the reassurance that Strong was seeking from him. In a letter sent from Liverpool on Friday, she described his note as kindly and said it was most welcome:

I shall now derive more benefit from my change and hope to return to my work in a more healthy frame of mind than that in which I left it. I fancy molehills were becoming mountains to me.

There are another two letters in the series, which record another attempt to resign by Strong – which again she later withdrew, although she did eventually resign in 1885.

In January 1883, she wrote to Macewen, referring to Mr McEwen who was chairman of the board of governors at Glasgow Royal Infirmary:

Nothing fresh has occurred. If Mr McEwen is left quite alone, I think his better judgement may come to the rescue. I did make a great mistake in saying – 'The conditions were such that I could not accept them'. I shall be very sorry to go now that the house is in good working order. I do not say it is perfect, but there is nothing more to bother me than you would find in any ordinary household.[8]

And in the following month she said:

I have seen Mr McEwen today. He was kindness itself and told me to write a letter to him to the effect that it was through a misapprehension my resignation was sent in, which I have done, & therefore you may look upon the matter as virtually settled.

I hope your throat is better. Thanking you for your kindness.[9]

It is believed only one letter from Macewen to Strong survives, written in 1884 when his work was attracting international attention and he had returned from addressing a major medical conference in Copenhagen. In it, he acknowledges the vital contribution of Strong and her nurses to his work, saying that she should share any honour which he is awarded:

My dear Mrs Strong, I have just returned from a trip in Norway .... I leave here for London tomorrow. We have not had rain since landing in Norway and the weather has been very hot ... You will be pleased to hear that I got a very hearty reception at the Congress of Copenhagen – it is a strange sound on the ear, the mingling of German 'hoch's' with the French and English sounds of applause – and as these burst forth when my name was mentioned to address the meeting, I confess I was a little put out ... I look on you and the nurses as part of myself and any honour which might be conferred on me is something which should be shared in by you.[10]

This was a letter which Strong had kept for forty years. She sent it to Macewen's family after his death in 1924 at the age of 75 with a note attached which read: 'The enclosed letter was received in the Royal Infirmary with extreme joy. We felt it showed an unusually appreciative nature and acted as a stimulant. One's efforts are by no means always acknowledged and this was a most generous acknowledgment.'

In his analysis, Gibson said it would be easy to read 'too much starry-eyed romanticism between the lines' in the relationship between Strong and Macewen. But he concluded:

There is no doubt of the affection between the two but equally no doubt that they invariably behaved to each other with complete propriety. It could be truer to regard their affection as based on a thorough appreciation and respect for the brilliance of each other and the rest of their story supports this.

Chapter Nine

Later Life: Travel, the Blitz and an OBE

In the years after she retired as matron from Glasgow Royal Infirmary, as we have seen, Strong continued her involvement with the nursing world, particularly when she moved back to Scotland from near Ruthin, where she had lived with her sister for a time before her sibling's death.

In 1926, when she was in her late seventies, she became involved as one of the founders of the British College of Nurses, an academic institution designed to provide nurses with a college where they could study for postgraduate qualifications. Strong was a supporter of Ethel Gordon Fenwick, also known as Mrs Bedford Fenwick, who spent decades campaigning for the state registration of nurses and had set up the college:

> As a loyal supporter of Mrs Bedford Fenwick, Mrs Strong threw her influence behind the British College of Nurses. She encouraged members of the Scottish Nurses Association to join and she addressed meetings of nurses explaining what the role of the College would be, providing postgraduate courses for nurses with scholarships and bursaries.[1]

The first diploma day was held in April 1927, when founder fellows were presented with certificates decorated with names recognising those who had made an outstanding contribution to nursing, which included Strong. She made a speech at the ceremony in which she said the college provided opportunities for postgraduate education for nurses beyond that provided by hospitals.[2] Once again this gives insight into Strong's belief that education should not stop and the profession is one of constant learning.

She also believed that her young nurses should not only study to become efficient in their duties but find 'strength and refreshment' in reading the great classics of literature. She held informal meetings where the works of authors such as Robert Browning and Thomas Carlyle were discussed.[3] For example, addressing the Glasgow Royal Infirmary Nurses' Reunion Dinner in 1922, she urged the audience to give a thought to the words of writer Joseph Conrad when he spoke of 'the consciousness of the worth and force of inner life' – which she characterised as individuality:

> This was the thought she wished the nurses to take away, and it would shape all their actions and create an atmosphere which would envelop them and give them a personality. Work could be noble or ignoble, just as the individual made it. Much strenuous work was needed, she said, before were brought to the perfect life, and no one need expect to attain more than that.[4]

For many years, Strong was involved with the RBNA and was a popular figure, particularly among younger members. When she was elected as a vice president in 1926, it was said to be through the nominations from young members of the executive committee:

> There is no more popular visitor to the Club than she, and while we are in the habit of finding that the people, who are still in active work, seem to find companionship mostly in their own set, while the others follow their particular inclinations in this respect, the young folks, by common consent, absorb Mrs Strong into their own group, and it is a very usual occurrence to find her by the hall fire surrounded by a group of youngsters listening to her wise admonitions, given with a mixture of humour and tolerance, that proves very acceptable to her audience, or entering into the experiences and amusements of youth with as keen a zest as they; she was the first purchaser of a ticket for the dance on the 30th of last month. More than once we have heard the wish expressed that we may journey to life's evening time with that same fragrancy of personality which characterises this great pioneer of Nursing Education.[5]

In 1930, Strong moved home again, this time to Edinburgh where she lived for nearly a decade. During this time – unsurprisingly given her age – she was not as active in the nursing world, but contact continued with correspondence and visits. In 1935, an appearance at the Scottish Nurses' Club in Bath Street in Glasgow was reported with the headline '90-year-old Edinburgh Speaker at Meeting':

> Among the speakers ... on Saturday was Mrs Strong of Edinburgh, a former matron of Glasgow Royal Infirmary who is now over 90 years of age. The Marchioness of Ailsa presided. Mrs Strong addressed the members on the subject of the international memorial to Florence Nightingale. She explained that the memorial would not be merely something for people to look at, but would take the form of scholarships for nurses, and to enable members of the profession to carry on their magnificent work on behalf of suffering humanity.[6]

The following year, she spoke at the New Year's Day meeting at Glasgow Royal Infirmary – and used the occasion to call for better organisation in the profession:

> Mrs Strong, speaking with remarkable vigour for her years, read messages from former nurses of the Royal Infirmary, now in New York, Australia and Shanghai. The training they had received in Glasgow was being put to use in their new spheres of activity, the letters indicated. Mrs Strong declined the honour of having originated the scheme of training nurses in the Royal Infirmary, and stated that the credit was due to the medical staff, who obtained the sanction of the managers

to carry it out. Her job, she added, had been to find the pupils, and that had not involved many difficulties. Glasgow at that time was waiting for such a scheme, and the success of the work was due to the nurses themselves. They had now carried their knowledge to all parts of the world.

She urged young nurses to maintain what had been achieved for them. The nursing profession needed real organisation. A century ago, she concluded, the profession of medical men was as disorganised at the nursing profession was today.[7]

Meanwhile, a campaign was ongoing for Strong to be officially recognised for her work with an honour from the state, and several petitions were lodged on her behalf. There was, however, opposition from St Thomas' Hospital which Strong appeared to have sympathy with. In a letter to a friend in August 1938 she highlighted the system introduced in Glasgow Royal Infirmary had somewhat 'eclipsed' the training which had previously been undertaken by the London hospital:

After nearly 85 years since Miss Nightingale's memorable work in the Crimea, followed by her arrangement with St Thomas' Hospital for the reception of pupils … then in 1893 to be eclipsed by the Royal Infirmary of Glasgow introducing a system for the preliminary instruction of nurse students … with St Thomas' powerful influence, it would not sacrifice its prestige to any authority.[8]

But the persistence of her supporters paid off and she was awarded an OBE – the oldest recipient of an honour that year. This was announced at the New Year meeting of staff and managers of Glasgow Royal Infirmary. At the age of 96, this was to be her last public appearance and it could not have been a more fitting one – surrounded by admirers and friends, receiving recognition for all she had done for nursing. Once again, she appeared to be defying her advanced years when she addressed the meeting in a 'firm, clear voice' on the subject of the future of nurses' education and its place in the medical colleges.[9] She received a standing ovation when she walked on to the platform from the nurses present:

By their applause, the nurses signified their appreciation of the new status which she was instrumental in gaining for those in the profession by her work in starting in the Royal Infirmary in 1893 the first preliminary training school for nurses in the world.

Mrs Strong spoke firmly and clearly when she rose to acknowledge the complimentary remarks of the Lord Provost and Sir James Macfarlane and to thank the nurses for presenting her with a bouquet of pink carnations. 'The conferment of this honour by the King is a tribute to a great life of service,' said the Lord

Provost to Mrs Strong. 'By honouring you,' he added, 'His Majesty has honoured the entire profession of which you have been a worthy leader and member.'[10]

An 'unfortunate accident' prevented Strong from receiving her award at Buckingham Palace – so the Duke of Buccleuch instead visited her at home and presented her with the OBE.[11]

Her great love of travel is frequently noted in accounts of her life. After her retirement in 1907 at the age of 64, she still appeared at nurses' congresses internationally in Canada, Finland, Egypt and Palestine. She attended the Dublin Nursing Conference and Exhibition in 1913 as a representative of the Scottish Nurses' Association.[12] In October 1929, she went to the Nurses' Congress in Montreal, speaking at a dinner for graduates of Toronto General Hospital, where it was noted she 'charmed them all with her personality and reminiscences'.[13]

In 1927, when she was in her late seventies, she addressed a conference of the International Council of Nurses in Geneva, giving a closing address which she began by asking her 'old friends to excuse an old woman if she was prosy, as she was generally asleep at that time':

Referring to the progress being made in the Nursing World, she illustrated this by saying that when in 1891 the Preliminary Training was launched in connection with the Royal Infirmary Glasgow, of which she was at that time Matron, she wrote to many Matrons and received two answers. One wrote that she thought it would produce a pseudo-scientific nurse, and the second that she did not have that education herself and she did not think it was wanted.

Strong concluded by noting her observations on the nursing profession, from the distance of someone who was no longer actively involved:

> She was now standing apart from active service, like a sentinel upon a watch tower and her sympathies went out to the young nurses. No doubt there were improvements to hours and recreation, but she thought the nurses of the present day worked just as hard as their predecessors as they had to give so much time to study.[14]

At the age of 86 she attempted a trip to India and China – although one had to be abandoned.[15] And a year later, at the age of 87, she made a broadcast in New York which went out across America.[16]

Her sprightliness and continuing zest for life in her later years was often remarked upon, such as in this report from Glasgow's Lady Provost in January 1939:

> At the presentation of prizes to the nurses in the Royal Infirmary we met that wonderful old woman Mrs Rebecca Strong – the doyen of the nursing profession.

Aged 96, she trained under Florence Nightingale and was once matron of the Royal Infirmary. Despite her age, she made a speech that was interesting and fluent.

She would love to have gone on longer – and I'd have loved to hear her – but I saw someone pulling discreetly at her coat to let her know her time was up.

The more I see of women like her, the more I begin to realise age is only what you make it. Your body may grow old, but there's no need to sit back, defeated by the years, and let your mind grow old with it. Mrs Strong has kept her mind active and young. We must all try to follow her example.[17]

In 1939, Strong moved back to Glasgow and lived in the Hyndland area of the city's west end. But in March 1941 her home was partly destroyed by a bomb in a series of attacks across the city carried out by the Luftwaffe. The destruction on 13 and 14 March is commonly known as the Clydebank Blitz, due to the devastation of that district, with more than 600 people were killed across Glasgow over 2 days.

Reports note that she was then 'persuaded' to move to Chester to live with her great-nephew and his wife – and it is not hard to imagine how extremely reluctant she would have been to give up her independence. But she continued her links with Scotland, including speaking at the Scottish Nurses' Club in 1940, when she was 97 years old.

Her advice to the gathering was, 'Don't be too disappointed when you do not succeed right away with the things you want in life.' She also commented on the Second World War, another global conflict she witnessed in her lifetime.

> She declared that all history was a succession of battles. If there was more real understanding of right and wrong in the world the present conflict would soon end. There would always be some people who preferred evil to good, but when a real peace came again she hoped that a restraint would be put on the side of evil. That would be a bigger struggle than the actual war.[18]

In August 1943, Strong celebrated her hundredth birthday and spent it sitting in her favourite armchair, 'surrounded by flowers' and listening to messages sent to her from all over the country.[19] Not only did she receive the usual telegram from the King George VI but a personal handwritten message from his mother, Queen Mary, whom she had met several times. It read: 'To Mrs Strong, with best wishes on your hundredth birthday, Mary R.'

***

On her hundredth birthday, she was sent a message from the British College of Nurses, signed by president Ethel Gordon Fenwick, as reported in *The British Journal of Nursing*:

Mrs Strong, who was a great traveller, took an active interest in the organisation of the International Council of Nurses and attended many of its gatherings, where she was always a personage of great interest to her colleagues from many lands. The following telegram was sent to Mrs Strong from the British College of Nurses, Ltd, of which she was an early fellow: 'The Fellows and Members of the British College of Nurses Ltd desire to convey their affectionate greetings, gratitude, and admiration to their eminent colleague (Mrs Rebecca Strong OBE), on attaining her hundredth birthday and wish her all the happiness she deserves in return for the eminent services she has rendered to the Nursing Profession of which she is so well beloved a pioneer'.

Another message on her hundredth birthday came in the form of an illuminated address from the Nightingale Fellowship at St Thomas' Hospital in London, where Strong had begun her career. Describing her as a pioneer in nursing it read:

Your call to youth at the International Congress of Nurses in 1929 assures us that you were young in thought, and ever looking forward to planning our own day's enterprise, in that it shall extend to the frontiers of life and enlarge its opportunities for men, women and children of all nations.[20]

The occasion of her centenary was widely noted in the press – where she was described as 'the grand old lady' of the nursing profession.[21] Strong's connections with Florence Nightingale, achievements in the nursing world and adventures in later life providing ample material for some colourful reports, such as in the *Manchester Evening News*:[22]

Ruffles of limerick lace over a delicate wrist … a spreading black satin gown … blue eyes wearing the wisdom of 100 years all but three days … thus one of Florence Nightingale's first nurses held court at Vicar's Cross, Chester, today. She will reach her centenary on Monday – Mrs Rebecca Strong, trusted colleague of the Lady of the Lamp, and she gave me this one philosophy from her journey through the years as she sat in her straight-backed chair with faintly powdered cheeks: 'Life is a struggle from beginning to end. The moment we stop struggling for better things there is death.'

Widowed at 24, this frail pioneer went around the London hospitals, thinking to become nurse. 'But they only wanted scrubbers,' she said. 'I wanted to be a nurse.'

So she gave up the idea – until she saw an advertisement in a magazine stating that Florence Nightingale wanted nurses. So she went to St Thomas's Hospital, to the school of Florence Nightingale, of whom she said today: 'She was a fine woman – and a good-looking woman, for her mind made her face. Florence Nightingale was never discouraging.' Nurse Rebecca Strong became the first nurse ever to take a temperature and was roundly rebuked for undertaking a doctor's prerogative.

The report noted she was one of five nurses chosen by the 'Lady of the Lamp' to carry out her work and had been matron of Dundee Infirmary and Glasgow Royal Infirmary, but she has also 'travelled all over the world and seen much':

She has seen Mussolini, and the shrewd old lady did not think much of him, for he arrived late for the soirée and was very abrupt. She has friends all over the world. Mrs Strong, who says, 'I am only an old-fashioned woman,' and a letter of congratulation in the handwriting of Queen Mary, with a signed photograph, has just arrived at the house where she is living with her great-nephew. Women today have wonderful advantages,' said the centenarian. 'And nurses study today things that only doctors knew in my day. There is every sign of even greater things ahead for the nursing profession.' Meanwhile she [fi]nds it is just amusing to be 100.

Another newspaper account showed how celebrating her hundredth year had been a busy time for Strong, who was still keeping active:

Mrs Rebecca Strong, who is living with her great-nephew Dr Charles J. Tisdale at Heathfield Vicar's Cross, Chester, will celebrate her 100th birthday on

Monday. She is one of the pioneers of modern nursing, being one of Miss Florence Nightingale's probationers at St Thomas's Hospital London. Later she was chosen by Miss Nightingale to inaugurate a new nursing scheme at Netley Military Hospital. Mrs Strong has had a busy week preparing for her birthday. She has been giving Press interviews and having her photograph taken. Today (Friday) she is doing a recording for the BBC who hope to include her talk in one of the Scottish bulletins. At the age of 31 she was appointed Matron of Dundee Infirmary. In 1879 she became Matron of Glasgow Royal Infirmary and, apart for one spell, remained in that post until 1907 when she retired. She claims the distinction of being the first nurse to take a temperature and recall with a chuckle that this audacious act earned her a reprimand for in those days nurses were only given menial tasks. It is a long cry from those far-off days to 1941 when Mrs Strong was bombed out of her Glasgow home – that was why she came to Chester. On New Year's Day 1939 she was awarded the OBE for her distinguished services to nursing and she celebrated the announcement by addressing a meeting of managers and nurses of Glasgow Royal Infirmary. She is still active and spends most of her spare time knitting comforts for members of the Forces.[23]

The BBC recorded a message from her to old friends and to younger nurses, which was broadcast on the radio. In November of that year, she also sent a message to be read at a screening of the 'The Lamp Still Burns', a film which follows a woman architect who changes careers to become a nurse, showing the demands of the job and raising the issue of better treatment of nurses. Even after turning 100, Strong was continuing to engage with the ongoing debates around the profession – and encouraging others to follow in her footsteps:

> I congratulate the modern nurse on living in a time of scientific and standardised progress. The basic ideas of nursing, however, do not change, and I would say to anyone embarking on a nursing career, that she is entering a noble calling indeed the most noble that any woman can take up. The work is strenuous and often exciting, but always well worth some sacrifice, and from now on many of the old and somewhat Spartan conditions of service will disappear, and I trust that the nurses' work in future will be eased of much of its hardship. If these few words of mine should encourage any waverer to take up nursing as her vocation, she may regard her decision as in some degree influenced by Florence Nightingale herself, as I do but pass on the inspiration which I received direct from the Lady of the Lamp, whom I am proud to have known.[24]

This was echoed in comments made by her great-nephew, Dr Charles Tisdale, who said that his aunt had shown a great interest in the Rushcliffe Report published in 1943, which made recommendations on issues such as salaries for nurses, educational grants and conditions for service in English hospitals. While he said the report had embodied many of her ideals for the profession, he added:

> But she has a dread of the profession becoming too standardised in the way of working hours and remuneration. It is also a horrible idea to her that, owning to war conditions, women should be 'directed' into nursing. She reads it as essentially a vocation to which one is called.[25]

In her later years, an accident to her thigh made it 'impossible for her to leave her chair without help' – but she was active in body and mind otherwise. Strong died on 24 April 1944, in Chester and was still knitting for the forces up to a week or two beforehand.[26] She left a personal estate of £5,843[27] – the equivalent of around £300,000 today. What is believed to be the last letter written by her, which is still in existence today, was a reply in response to congratulations from Glasgow Royal Infirmary physician Dr David Smith on reaching her hundredth birthday. In clear handwriting she wrote:

> I am grateful for your kind congratulations on my hundredth birthday – it was a very happy one, surrounded with numerous tokens of sweet remembrance – and I was able to join in a most sumptuous tea. Think the Minister of Food might not have approved. The dear old GRI is never long out of my thoughts – as always glad to hear of it.[28]

Chapter Ten

Legacy: 'The Pupil Should Surpass the Teacher'

How best to sum up the many achievements of Rebecca Strong? For one she was instrumental in helping move the nursing professions from the days of the fictional Mrs Gamp into an organised, educated and professional workforce. Her vision and determination saw the introduction of a system which changed the face of nursing and as testament to its success, still forms the basis of the block training which staff undergo today. No mean achievement for a woman who was left a single mother in her twenties and decided to train as a nurse when it was not seen as a respectable profession:

> Her decision to train in a hospital, rather than practise nursing among the poor of her neighbourhood as many widows did, involved separation from her daughter who can only have been three or four years old at the time. Again, by choosing the Nightingale School when Miss Nightingale was still a national hero and the school an experiment showed spirit and later, her decision to leave Netley Hospital, contradicting the orders of Miss Nightingale and Mrs Wardroper, was

the act of an independent person. It is significant that it was in Scotland that Mrs Strong was able to fulfil her potential. It would have been unusual for a woman with her working-class background to have been appointed matron of a large voluntary hospital in England.[1]

Yet when writing about her own life, Strong was characteristically modest about her achievements. Her short memoirs published in 1935, when she was in her late eighties, starts:

It has often been suggested to me to give the story of my nursing life, but I hesitate to do so, as it seems to me almost impossible for anyone to write impartially of themselves. One's own little bit is very insignificant when compared with the multitude of women who have freely given their lives not merely to nursing, but to the other branches of work concerning the welfare of the Empire. I am not thinking of the noble deeds and sacrifices called forth by the awful war (extraordinary circumstances produce extraordinary action), but of those who are scattered over the world working steadily on from day to day in obscure corners under the most adverse conditions, and little heard of them. Nurses working in our slums and Highlands and similar places in distant lands can tell stirring tales of want of material and appliances, and sometimes without medical aid, travelling long distances under trying conditions of rail, road and boat. I have met with many such. Anyone acquainted with nurses, and encouraging fireside talks, will hear many a heroic tale, told with simplicity and unconsciousness of doing anything unusual or worthy of comment. These are true missionaries in the best sense of the word.[2]

Strong also summarised her own advice to nurses in publications, including 'Hints to Beginners in the Work of Nursing', published by James C. Erskine in 1882 for 'private circulation', which covered a wide range of topics. It begins with an outline of the ideal characteristics for a nurse:

> Qualities to be cultivated by those desirous of devoting themselves to this work – Truthfulness, cleanliness, observation, accuracy, punctuality, order, obedience, gentleness with firmness, a pleasant voice and manner. At first mention of truthfulness some may be apt to take offence. You do not need to do this, as thorough 'transparent truthfulness' is most difficult to acquire. It means a certain amount of moral courage in not sparing one's errors, as well as the power of representing things as they are – uncoloured by imagination.

She went on to underline the importance of cleanliness, including 'effectual out-of-sight cleanliness' which is not so easily achieved, before addressing the need to be able to take responsibility for patients and make detailed observations:

No-one knows so well as a doctor the changes which are likely to take place during the intervals of his visits; and if you realise your responsibility in being left with a patient during those intervals, and know how much the treatment depends on your report, I am sure you will take care that there shall be no vagueness in the giving of said report. Take the question of food. A good nurse should be able to state definitely the quantity of food taken in either ounces or pints. This can be easily managed by measuring a certain quantity, if liquid, and noting it down; and when finished, repeat. I do not mean you to have it constantly beside the patient, but set aside. If solid food, you should accustom yourself to the judging of quantities by ounces – I am not speaking of convalescent patients, but the very sick. Sleep should also be carefully noted, the length of each sleep, whether restlessness is more marked before 12 or after – muttering or restless sleep. It is sometimes very difficult to distinguish between sleep and unconsciousness; but still, a careful observant nurse will be able in time to acquire the necessary knowledge.

However, Strong warned that the role of the nurse is to 'carry out instructions' and not treat patients according to their own ideas. But she said this should not be a 'blind' but a 'watchful' intelligence. Another necessity she outlined is the need to gain the confidence of patients, which she says would not be accomplished by either 'harsh rule' or 'foolish indulgence':

A quiet unobtrusive self-possession will do much towards gaining this confidence … If your patient's mind is kept in a tranquil condition, it will do much towards the recovery of his body. A loud clumsy nurse will certainly never succeed in gaining this tranquillity for her patients. If a patient finds himself to be in the hands of a nurse who has his sole interest and welfare at heart, it is almost miraculous to find how thoroughly she is trusted and obeyed. Let her be a nurse in name only – without the true spirit – and most assuredly her patients will know it almost at the first touch and word.

She also emphasised a theme which she frequently referred to in her nursing and teaching work – that any training and education undertaken is only the beginning of learning for nurses:

A nurse must, to a great extent, be her own teacher. The most that can be done in the way of direct teaching, is to give a few general principles, which may guide you in your observations of the sick, and you must make these the foundation of your work. As to turning out a complete nurse, one who has mastered all the intricacies of her work – that is an impossibility; you must be ever learning. Each physician and surgeon has his own particular manner of working, and a nurse must remember it is her duty to learn these ways, and not suppose there is only one way of working.

Another point she made is that nurses must have to use their own judgement, giving this practical advice, for example, on the feeding of patients:

> Take bread as an example – the first thing to be done is to look round your ward, and consider the number of sick people you have who cannot take thickly cut bread and butter, but would enjoy a thin slice neatly served. One small piece thoroughly enjoyed will do your patient more good than a larger amount taken without any relish. Always cut less than will be required for a meal, it is easy to cut more; and cut bread cannot possibly be kept moist, and used with any degree of comfort for the next meal.

She concluded:

> The foregoing remarks are nothing more than is already intimated, 'Hints'; and if they lead you to think about your work, and are any help to you in directing your thoughts, my object will be attained.

Strong's advice is also preserved in a publication of her lecture given at Glasgow Royal Infirmary in 1893, on 'Introductory Remarks to Practical Classes on Ward Work'. She began by quoting the late Sir James Simpson, a renowned Scottish doctor who pioneered advances in areas including obstetrics and anaesthesia, on advice which he gave to students: 'Your aim is, as far as possible, to alleviate human suffering, to gladden, as well as to prolong, the course of human life.'

She outlined what she believed were the required characteristics for nursing as follows:

> The first requisite is sound health with a well-regulated mind, whose equilibrium is not easily lost; undue nervousness and sensitiveness are fatal, they must be conquered, or at least kept in subjection. Quickness of hearing and sight are desirable; where there is the least defect of sight, allow no false sentiment to deter you from the constant use of glasses. There is no Royal road to nursing any more than any other calling. People speak of born nurses. Granted, that some have a natural aptitude for nursing, as for other professions, but it must be cultivated.

Strong observed that nursing is not 'mechanical work' for which 'hard and fast rules' can be given, even to trainees:

> It is an ever-varying work, each Physician and Surgeon bringing the results of his own particular studies to bear upon the individual patient; therefore, keep an open mind, guard against taking too narrow a view of things, thinking your own little bit of knowledge is conclusive. Nursing, like all other arts, is progressive; the facts of today will yield to the knowledge of tomorrow. Nothing human is final, all knowledge is

cumulative, and upon the foundation you receive now, build up a superstructure which shall help on the ages yet to come. The pupil should surpass the teacher. The teacher but passes on the knowledge which has been gathered from the past and the present; it is for you to add to those venerable piles of learning.

She cautioned of the difficulties of the work saying that 'very much that is unpleasant will fall to your lot', but went on:

The woman who shrinks from this had better pause at the threshold of her career and consider how far she is prepared to subdue self and work only for the good of others. Our poorer and less fortunately placed brethren with whom you will now come into contact have not had your advantages, and must be dealt with in a loving and helpful spirit. Any superciliousness on your part will be keenly felt by them and resented. Meet them as fellow creatures, not as inferior beings, remembering that it is a mere accident of birth and not any personal merit of your own, which has placed you in different circumstances.

However, she also went on to describe the joys of the job as follows:

There is much, on the other hand, to render the life an attractive one. You are not dealing with machines, but living beings in whom there is a responsive chord which is often wonderfully touched by a sympathetic feeling, not an undue obtrusive show of feeling which is harmful, but the heartfelt touch of sorrow for another's affliction which produces the gentle touch and word.

She concluded the lecture with the following thoughts:

The education received at school is only a foundation for the real education of life. If you have received only the education of the parrot, a mere repeating of certain formulae by rote, it will be of little service to you, quickly falling away, and leaving you a barren soil; on the other hand, if you have been taught to think, and weigh well whatever is placed before you, deducting your own conclusions, then you will have a storehouse of wealth from which you can continually draw, and all subjects will be food for thought. I want you to understand that you must, to a great extent, be your own teachers.

The contribution of Strong was recognised not only by Macewen but by his family following his death in 1924. In 1942, his son, who was a surgeon at Glasgow Royal Infirmary, decide to mark the fiftieth anniversary of the first lectures being given to nurses at the hospital by commissioning two medals which were to be awarded annually in recognition of the work of his father and Strong.

One featuring a bust of his father was to be awarded to the best practical surgical nurse in her year and one with the bust of Strong to be given to the best practical medical nurse in the year. Strong welcomed the idea which came at a time when she was struggling with her health and wrote in January 1942 to the Macewen family: 'It was nice to hear even your name, having suffered much from depression the old name is like a bit of inspiration putting fresh life into me.'[3]

And in another letter in February of that year she stated:

Your letter is invaluable in helping to raise me out of my desponding condition and perverted view of things, it is deplorable, treatment for anaemia of the brain is still going on, my own opinion is that it is old age – ninety-nine in August.[4]

The first medal ceremony was held in January 1943:

When the nurses' prize-giving ceremony took place recently at Glasgow Royal Infirmary, two new awards were made for the first time. These are the Macewen Medal for Surgical Nursing and the Mrs Strong Medal for Medical Nursing. The medals were given in each case for the best practical surgical and medical nursing, and the accent in on the 'practical', which includes aspects of the profession possibly not found in the text-books, such as cheerfulness – and so on. Mr J.A.C. Macewen, honorary consulting surgeon to the Royal Infirmary, and son of the late Sir William Macewen, is presenting both medals, which are to be awarded annually. The medal for medical nursing has been designed by Miss Ivy Gardner, a Glasgow sculptor, and a drawing of the design is in the Fine Art Institute. On the one side is a head of Mrs Rebecca Strong OBE, a former distinguished Matron of the Royal Infirmary, now enjoying well-earned retirement, and on the other an inscription indicating the purpose of the award. Mrs Strong is now in her hundredth year, and we wish her all the good health possible.

Strong was also a firm supporter of women's suffrage and of equality in education. Her career was not always a happy one – the first stint as matron at Glasgow Royal Infirmary came with huge challenges and placed a strain on her health. But in a lesson in perseverance, when she returned it was to enjoy one of the happiest times of her life. She was always keen to follow new developments in training and education, following her own advice to younger generations to keep an open mind. Despite all this, her reputation as a pioneer in nursing education is said to have received greater recognition in North American than in Britain.[5]

Yet within the nursing world, her contribution was acknowledged and praised. In an article, 'Nurses of Note', published in *The British Journal of Nursing* in 1924, it was summed up:

The influence of Mrs Strong on the development
of nursing extends far beyond her work at the Royal
Infirmary, and her wonderful vitality was demonstrated
in her speech at the recent reunion of the Glasgow Royal
Infirmary Nurses, when she counselled the members of
the League to be true to the best that is in them. A staunch
supporter of the movement for State Registration of
Nurses, Mrs Strong did much to promote its attainment
through the weary years of opposition, and as President
of the Scottish Nurses' Association, [she was] a forceful,
inspiring influence in the Nursing Profession. The
Nursing Profession, both now and in the future, should
offer thanks for the self-denial, the energy, the altruism,
and the devotion to the public interest which, under
Mrs Strong's leadership, made the training at the Royal
Infirmary, Glasgow, second to none in the kingdom and
have made her name honoured, not only by the Nursing
Profession in her own country, but throughout the world.[6]

Another insight into why she was so acclaimed as a nurse
comes from a report published many years after her death
on a prize-giving ceremony at North Staffordshire Royal
Infirmary. Sir Arthur Tomson, a hospital board and General
Medical Council member is quoted as saying of Strong:

She used to look after five wards, and sat on the staircase
to hear where the cries came from. There are subjects in

which exams are a reliable test, but the qualities needed for a nurse, like compassion and a desire to serve, are immeasurable by examination.[7]

Her death was described as the 'passing of a great pioneer' in a letter of tribute which was published shortly after her death[8] and praises her 'courageous and unwavering fight for the dignity and the rights of the nurse':

> We have read and heard much of Mrs. Strong's wonderful life for the profession of nursing. She carried the Nightingale tradition to Scotland, and was an eloquent and shining example of its inspiration. I heard from her own lips a witty and spirited account of her determined efforts for better conditions and it was from a money point of view, a sacrifice to return to the Royal Infirmary. What a triumph, and what an opportunity which she grasped with both hands!

One of Strong's most famous quotes was, 'I'm afraid I was a rather troublesome woman.' Having examined her battles and successes, it is hard to imagine her saying this without a mischievous glint in her eye. Looking back on her long and remarkable life, these words should not be viewed as an apology but a celebration of her ability to challenge the status quo and authority, resulting in achievements in the nursing profession which have made a lasting impact and deserve to be remembered for years to come.

Acknowledgements

With grateful thanks to everyone who has helped with this book, particularly the staff at the following for their assistance with research:

Friends of Glasgow Royal Infirmary
Glasgow Royal Infirmary Medical Illustration Services
Royal College of Nursing Archives
Royal College of Physicians and Surgeons of Glasgow

Select Bibliography

Baly, Monica, *Florence Nightingale and the Nursing Legacy* (Wiley–Blackwell, 1997)

Dickens, Charles, *Martin Chuzzlewit* (Penguin Classics, 2000)

Dingwall, Helen, *A History of Scottish Medicine: Themes and Influences* (Edinburgh University Press, 2003)

Henderson, Mary, *Dundee Women's Trail* (Dundee Women's Trail, 2008)

Jenkinson, Jacqueline, Moss, Michael, and Russell, Iain, *The Royal: The History of Glasgow Royal Infirmary, 1794–1994* (Published by the Bicentenary Committee on behalf of Glasgow Royal Infirmary NHS Trust, 1994)

Lynch, Michael, *Oxford Companion to Scottish History* (Oxford University Press, 2011)

Macdonald, Fiona, *Dundee A Very Peculiar History* (Scribblers, 2015)

McGann, Susan, *The Battle of the Nurses* (Scutari Press, 1992)

End Notes

Introduction: 'A Very Troublesome Woman'

1. YouTube, Friends of GRI, *Museum Opening Event May 31st 2022*: www.youtube.com/watch?v=2gtpPj1321M
2. *The Herald,* 22 May 2021
3. *Glasgow Herald*, 20 August 1943
4. *Comprehensive Child and Adolescent Nursing*, 'Celebrating the Contribution of Florence Nightingale to Contemporary Nursing', Glasper, Edward Alan, 2020, 43:4, 233–239, DOI: 10.1080/24694193.2020.1824256

Chapter One: Old, Weak, Drunken, Stupid: The Stereotype of Early Nurses

1. *Martin Chuzzlewit*, Charles Dickens, Penguin edition, 2000, p.303
2. *The Nursing Record and Hospital World*, 26 September 1896, p.253
3. Ibid., p.254
4. Ibid.
5. *The British Journal of Nursing,* Volume 29 Issue 13, 'Celebrating Florence Nightingale and her Contribution to Nursing', Glasper, Professor Alan
6. *Nurse Janet Porter – nursing at the RIE before the 'Nightingale takeover'* – lhsa.blogspot.com/2022/08/nurse-janet-porter-nursing-at-rie.html

7. Ibid.
8. *Florence Nightingale and the Nursing Legacy*, Monica Baly, Wiley, 1999, p.viii
9. Ibid., p.ix
10. Ibid.
11. *Comprehensive Child and Adolescent Nursing*, 'Celebrating the Contribution of Florence Nightingale to Contemporary Nursing', Glasper
12. Ibid.
13. *Journal of Infection Prevention*, 'Revisiting Florence Nightingale: International Year of the Nurse and Midwife 2020'. Loveday H.P., 2020;21(1):4–6. doi:10.1177/1757177419896246
14. *Notes on Nursing*, Florence Nightingale, p.11
15. *Comprehensive Child and Adolescent Nursing*, 'Celebrating the Contribution of Florence Nightingale to Contemporary Nursing', Glasper
16. *The Nursing Record and Hospital World*, 24 June 1899, p.494
17. *Comprehensive Child and Adolescent Nursing*, 'Celebrating the Contribution of Florence Nightingale to Contemporary Nursing', Glasper

Chapter Two: Learning from Florence Nightingale

1. *Midwife, Health Visitor & Community Nurse*, December 1974, 'Distinguished British Nurses of the Past: Mrs Rebecca Strong', p.395
2. *The Battle of the Nurses: a study of eight women who have influenced the development of professional nursing 1880–1930*, Susan McGann, Scutari Press, 1992, p.103
3. YouTube, Friends of GRI, *Rebecca Strong – 'a troublesome woman'*: www.youtube.com/watch?v=8u-Y_1_UKUM
4. Ibid.

5. Ibid.
6. *The British Journal of Nursing*, January 1924, p.3
7. *Reminiscences*, Rebecca Strong, Douglas & Foulis, 1935, p.5
8. *The British Journal of Nursing*, January 1924, p.3
9. *Reminiscences*, Strong, p.6
10. *Florence the Women*, Florence Nightingale Museum, www.florence-nightingale.co.uk/kaiserwerth/
11. *Reminiscences*, Strong, p.7
12. *The Battle of the Nurses*, McGann, p.105
13. *Midwife, Health Visitor & Community Nurse*, December 1974, 'Distinguished British Nurses of the Past: Mrs Rebecca Strong', p.396
14. *The Era*, 9 May 1869 – www.netley-military-cemetery.co.uk/1864–1900-early-life-at-the-hospital
15. www.netley-military-cemetery.co.uk/1864–1900-early-life-at-the-hospital/
16. *The Battle of the Nurses*, McGann, p.104
17. *The Nursing Record and Hospital World*, 4 January 1902

Chapter Three: Raising the Status of Nurses in Dundee

1. *Dundee Courier*, 24 January 1949
2. *Dundee Courier*, 1 January 1874
3. *Dundee Courier*, 10 March 1874
4. *Reminiscences*, Strong, p.10
5. *Spectra*, NHS Tayside staff magazine, issue 42 June–July 2009, p.8
6. *The Battle of the Nurses*, McGann, p.105
7. *Dundee Women's Trail*, published by Dundee Women's Trail, 2008, p.29
8. *Dundee Courier*, 15 June 1875

9. *Dundee Women's Trail*, p.31
10. *Dundee Courier and Argus*, 18 December 1876
11. *Dundee Courier*, 29 December 1874
12. *Dundee Courier*, 5 January 1877
13. *Dundee Evening Telegraph*, 10 December 1929
14. *The British Journal of Nursing*, January 1930, p.19
15. *The Evening Telegraph*, 29 May 1939
16. *Spectra*, NHS Tayside staff magazine, issue 42 June–July 2009, p.8

Chapter Four: A Turbulent Time at Glasgow Royal Infirmary

1. *The Battle of the Nurses*, McGann, p.105
2. *The History of the Glasgow Royal Infirmary 1974–1994*, Jacqueline Jenkinson, Michael Moss & Iain Russell, published by the Bicentenary Committee on behalf of Glasgow Royal Infirmary 1994, p.142
3. *Midwife, Health Visitor & Community Nurse*, December 1974, 'Distinguished British Nurses of the Past: Mrs Rebecca Strong', p.397
4. *The Battle of the Nurses*, McGann, p.105
5. *The History of the Glasgow Royal Infirmary 1974–1994*, Jenkinson, Moss & Russell, p.129
6. Ibid.
7. Ibid.
8. The Royal College of Physicians and Surgeons of Glasgow, letters from Rebecca Strong to William Macewen, 15 April and 28 August 1882
9. *The British Journal of Nursing*, January 1924
10. *The History of the Glasgow Royal Infirmary 1974–1994*, Jenkinson, Moss & Russell, p.129

11. *The Battle of the Nurses*, McGann, p.110
12. *North British Daily Mail*, 2 September 1891, p.4
13. Ibid.
14. *North British Daily Mail*, 3 September 1891
15. *The Nursing Record*, 1 October 1891, p.170
16. *The Nursing Record*, 15 October 1891, p.194
17. *The Battle of the Nurses*, McGann, p.110

Chapter Five: 'Setting Things Straight' in Glasgow

1. *Glasgow Medical Journal,* July 1944; 'Mrs. Rebecca Strong (née Thorogood), O.B.E. Pioneer in Nursing and Nursing Education', John Patrick. 142(1):8–11. PMCID: PMC5955648
2. *Reminiscences*, Strong, p.11
3. *The Nursing Record*, 5 November 1891
4. Ibid.
5. Ibid.
6. *Reminiscences*, Strong, p.11
7. *RCN Magazine,* 'Nursing history: the first male nurses', Dr Stuart Wildman, 29 April 2020
8. 'Our latest information about nursing and midwifery in the UK', Nursing and Midwifery Council, April 2021-September 2021
9. *The History of the Glasgow Royal Infirmary 1974–1994*, Jenkinson, Moss & Russell
10. *The Battle of the Nurses*, McGann, p.111

Chapter Six: The 'Art of Nursing' Begins

1. *The Battle of the Nurses*, McGann, p.111
2. *The Nursing Record*, 12 January 1893, p.21
3. 'Distinguished British Nurses of the Past: Mrs Rebecca Strong', p.397

4. *The British Journal of Nursing*, January 1924, p.3
5. *The Nursing Record and Hospital World*, 17 November 1894, p.330
6. *The Nursing Record and Hospital World*, 10 November 1984, p.311
7. *The Battle of the Nurses*, McGann, p.114
8. *The Nursing Record and Hospital World*, 31 August 1901
9. *The Nursing Record and Hospital World*, 19 October 1901
10. *The Battle of the Nurses*, McGann, p.115
11. *The Nursing Record and Hospital World*, 15 January 1898, p.53
12. *Coatbridge Leader*, 27 April 1907

Chapter Seven: Campaigning for Registration and a New Club for Nurses

1. *Morning Leader*, 10 July 1908
2. *Hampshire Chronicle*, 20 May 1905
3. *The Battle of the Nurses*, McGann, pp.116–117
4. Ibid.
5. *The British Journal of Nursing*, 5 June 1909, p.226
6. Ibid., p.227
7. Ibid.
8. *Hereford Times*, 15 May 1909
9. *The British Journal of Nursing*, 17 July 1909, p.56
10. *The Battle of the Nurses*, McGann, p.117
11. Ibid. p.119
12. *The British Journal of Nursing*, 8 July 1916, p.27
13. *The Battle of the Nurses*, McGann, p.120
14. *The British Journal of Nursing*, December 1926, p.277
15. *The NMC register 1 April 2022–31 March 2023*, published by the Nursing and Midwifery Council

16. *The Battle of the Nurses*, McGann, p.121
17. *The British Journal of Nursing*, 21 December 1918, p.386
18. *The British Journal of Nursing*, 4 January 1919, p.4
19. Ibid., p.5
20. *The Battle of the Nurses*, McGann, p.121

Chapter Eight: Dear William Macewen …

1. *The Herald*, 26 May 2019
2. *The Herald*, 22 May, 2021
3. *Mrs Rebecca Strong, Sir William Macewen and the First Nurses Preliminary Training School,* Tom Gibson, DSc, FRCS, Royal College of Physicians and Surgeons of Glasgow (RCPSG) archives
4. RCPSG archives letter 15 April 1882
5. Ibid., 28 August 1882
6. *The Battle of the Nurses*, McGann, p.108
7. RCPSG archives letter 17 November 1882
8. Ibid., 23 January 1883
9. Ibid., 7 February 1883
10. Ibid., 24 August 1884

Chapter Nine: Later Life: Travel, the Blitz and an OBE

1. *The Battle of the Nurses*, McGann, p.124
2. Ibid.
3. *Glasgow Medical Journal,* July 1944; 'Mrs. Rebecca Strong (née Thorogood), O.B.E. Pioneer in Nursing and Nursing Education', John Patrick. 142(1):8–11. PMCID: PMC5955648
4. *The British Journal of Nursing*, 30 December 1922, p.425
5. *The British Journal of Nursing*, November 1926, p.251

6. *Edinburgh Evening News*, 1 April 1935, p.5
7. *The Scotsman*, 2 January 1936, p.5
8. Ibid.
9. Ibid.
10. *The British Journal of Nursing*, February 1939, p.31
11. *Liverpool Daily Post*, 19 August 1943
12. *The British Journal of Nursing*, 26 April 1913, p.329
13. *The British Journal of Nursing*, October 1927, p.276
14. Ibid., p.237
15. *Glasgow Medical Journal*, July 1944; 'Mrs. Rebecca Strong (née Thorogood), O.B.E. Pioneer in Nursing and Nursing Education', John Patrick. 142(1):8–11. PMCID: PMC5955648
16. *The Chronicle*, 29 April 1944
17. *The Sunday Post*, 8 January 1939
18. *The Scotsman*, 1 April 1940, p.3
19. *Evening Express*, 23 August 1943, p.3
20. Ibid.
21. *Western Times*, 27 August 1943
22. *Manchester Evening News*, 19 August 1943
23. *The Chronicle*, 21 August 1943
24. *The Cheshire Observer*, 20 November 1943, p.6
25. *The Liverpool Echo*, 19 August 1943, p.3
26. *Aberdeen Press and Journal*, 26 April 1944
27. *Shields Daily News*, 31 July 1944, p.5
28. *Mrs Rebecca Strong*, Gibson, DSc, FRCS, Royal College of Physicians and Surgeons of Glasgow (RCPSG) archives

Chapter Ten: Legacy: 'The Pupil Should Surpass the Teacher'

1. *The Battle of the Nurses*, McGann, p.126
2. *Reminiscences*, Strong, pp.3–44

3. *The Battle of the Nurses*, McGann, p.125
4. Ibid.
5. Ibid., p.128
6. *The British Journal of Nursing*, January 1924, p.3
7. *Evening Sentinel*, 10 April 1963, p.4
8. *The British Journal of Nursing*, May 1944, p.59

Index